Rec

D0705887

Using Technology in
Dementia Care

by the same author

Adaptive Interaction and Dementia
How to Communicate without Speech
Dr Maggie Ellis and Professor Arlene Astell
Illustrated by Suzanne Scott
ISBN 978 1 78592 197 1
eISBN 978 1 78450 471 7

of related interest

**Sharing Sensory Stories and Conversations
with People with Dementia**
A Practical Guide
Joanna Grace
ISBN 978 1 78592 409 5
eISBN 978 1 78450 769 5

**A Creative Toolkit for Communication
in Dementia Care**
Karrie Marshall
ISBN 978 1 84905 694 6
eISBN 978 1 78450 206 5

Young Onset Dementia
A Guide to Recognition, Diagnosis, and Supporting
Individuals with Dementia and Their Families
Hilda Hayo, Alison Ward, and Jacqueline Parkes
Foreword by Wendy Mitchell
ISBN 978 1 78592 117 9
eISBN 978 1 78450 383 3

Using Technology in Dementia Care

A Guide to Technology Solutions for Everyday Living

Edited by PROFESSOR ARLENE ASTELL,
DR SARAH KATE SMITH and DR PHIL JODDRELL

Jessica Kingsley *Publishers*
London and Philadelphia

First published in 2019
by Jessica Kingsley Publishers
73 Collier Street
London N1 9BE, UK
and
400 Market Street, Suite 400
Philadelphia, PA 19106, USA

www.jkp.com

Copyright © Jessica Kingsley Publishers 2019

Front cover image source: Shutterstock®.

All rights reserved. No part of this publication may be reproduced in any
material form (including photocopying, storing in any medium by electronic
means or transmitting) without the written permission of the copyright owner
except in accordance with the provisions of the law or under terms of a licence
issued in the UK by the Copyright Licensing Agency Ltd. www.cla.co.uk or in
overseas territories by the relevant reproduction rights organisation, for details
see www.ifrro.org. Applications for the copyright owner's written permission to
reproduce any part of this publication should be addressed to the publisher.

Warning: The doing of an unauthorised act in relation to a copyright work
may result in both a civil claim for damages and criminal prosecution.

Library of Congress Cataloging in Publication Data
A CIP catalog record for this book is available from the Library of Congress

British Library Cataloguing in Publication Data
A CIP catalogue record for this book is available from the British Library

ISBN 978 1 78592 417 0
eISBN 978 1 78450 779 4

Printed and bound in Great Britain

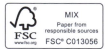

MIX
Paper from
responsible sources
FSC® C013056

Contents

Preface

Welcome to *Using Technology in Dementia Care: A Guide to Technology Solutions for Everyday Living.* This book combines up-to-date knowledge about technology for dementia, with examples of currently available technology and guidance on how to select and adopt technologies for dementia, with the experiences of people living with dementia. We decided to write this book because we recognised the need for a common-sense guide to help people with dementia and their care partners navigate the increasingly complex world of technology. We believe this book is timely as the numbers of people living with dementia are growing, creating rising demand for care and support. Given the current lack of drug treatments for dementia and rising numbers of people needing care, the potential of technology is increasingly being recognised. The past 20 years have seen a wide range of technological innovations developed, including those that address the needs of people with dementia to continue activities of daily life, and maintain physical, social and recreational activity and communication with caregivers. Technology has also been applied to addressing the needs of caregivers both at home and in care settings for education, support, safety and security. Indeed, much of the research has focused on the needs of caregivers and this book includes examination of the main developments in this area.

The many and varied developments in technology for dementia include both hardware (devices) and software (applications, programmes and services), including off-the-shelf technologies such as computers, smartphones, Global Positioning Systems (GPS), sensors and motion-detection systems. There have also been items created especially for dementia, including software applications, wayfinding devices and robots. However, there is currently a lack of public knowledge about the availability of technology for dementia as well as confusion created by aggressive advertising, particularly of applications that can allegedly prevent dementia. Additionally, the rapidly increasing availability of commercial products, such as smartphones and tablets, has created a need for accessible information and guidance for seeking out technologies that have been demonstrated to be useful. Once identified, most people also need guidance on how to incorporate devices and applications into their lives. This requires behaviour change to learn how to use new devices, start using them and make space in our busy lives to use them regularly and as recommended.

This book summarises current research knowledge about technology for dementia and presents practical information on identifying when a technology could be helpful, simple tips to choose appropriate items and guidance on how to introduce them into daily life. It also covers some basic information on common obstacles and barriers to technology, things to keep in mind when using technology, and making the most of what is available. In addition, people living with dementia share their practical experiences of using technology in their everyday lives. We hope you find their insights and the other information contained in *Using Technology in Dementia Care: A Guide to Technology Solutions for Everyday Living* interesting and useful.

PART 1

An Overview of Technology for Dementia

Chapter 1

An Introduction to Technology for Dementia

Professor Arlene Astell, *Professor of Neurocognitive Disorders,*
University of Reading, UK, and Research Chair in Dementia,
Ontario Shores Centre for Mental Health Sciences, Canada

Erica Dove, *Research Assistant,*
Ontario Shores Centre for Mental Health Sciences, Canada

Dr Alexandra Hernandez, *Postdoctoral Researcher,*
Ontario Shores Centre for Mental Health Sciences, Canada

Introduction

The advent of smartphones and tablets in the past ten years has opened up personal computing to many new audiences and with it created increasing interest in how such devices can be used to empower people. Similarly, growing awareness and availability of emerging technologies such as virtual reality (VR), robots, smart home systems (e.g. Amazon Alexa, Google Home Hub) and autonomous (i.e. driverless) vehicles are causing an explosion of interest in how they can improve wellbeing, including for those living with dementia. Although it has only recently gained mainstream attention, research into applying technology to dementia has been taking place alongside biomedical research for many decades. This chapter highlights the main focus of technological research in relation to people living with dementia, family caregivers and organisations that support people living with dementia.

Before examining the ways in which technology has been applied to empower people living with dementia, however, it is important to briefly highlight the types of difficulties they face. As is well known, dementia is an umbrella term applied to a number of illnesses and conditions that cause progressive, irreversible decline in cognitive function. The most common cause of dementia is Alzheimer's disease (AD), which is characterised by gradual inability to form new memories. This means individuals have better recollection for people and events from the past than the present and face difficulty learning new information. Age is the biggest risk factor for AD and although dementia is considered to be an age-related condition, there are several dementia subtypes, including frontotemporal dementia (FTD), primary progressive aphasia (PPA) and posterior cortical atrophy (PCA), that are more common in people in their fifties and sixties.

One thing that makes developing interventions for dementia extremely difficult is that each dementia subtype has a unique cognitive and behavioural profile. These are all defined in the *Diagnostic and Statistical Manual* (American Psychiatric Association 2013) under the heading 'major neurocognitive disorders', where the different effects on cognition and behaviour are described. This means that people with different types of dementia face different types of challenges in their everyday lives. FTD, for example, has two variants – frontal and temporal – with frontal-variant characterised more by changes in behaviour than cognition, including disinhibition, risk taking and lack of empathy. The temporal-variant of FTD, also known as semantic dementia, is notable for the loss of the ability to recognise items (e.g. everyday implements) and the meanings of words. In addition, there are three variants of PPA, all of which affect language in separate and distinct ways and which have a major impact on communication, social interaction and relationships. PCA, on the other hand, primarily affects the processing of visual information, resulting in problems with navigation, spatial orientation and driving. Understanding the extensive range of cognitive and behavioural effects of different dementia types highlights the breadth of the challenges people with dementia face, and how these interfere with different aspects of their lives and require a comprehensive range of solutions.

As there are currently no disease-modifying drug therapies for any dementia subtypes and little drug discovery research into the less common ones, there is huge potential for technology, in the forms of devices, applications and services, to assess and optimise the functioning of people who live with dementia (Smith 2013). In addition, technology can benefit families caring for a relative with dementia through dedicated devices and services, plus support through online forums and education about dementia. Technology can also support service providers through a digitally enabled workforce, assessment and monitoring functions, and provision of interventions. These are further explored in the other chapters of this book. To date a wide range of technologies has been applied to an equally wide range of challenges created by dementia, which is summarised below (see also Joddrell and Astell 2016; Lorenz *et al.* 2017; Meiland *et al.* 2017 for recent literature reviews).

Research areas of technology for dementia

Assessment

One of the major ways in which technology has been applied has been to develop new ways of conducting assessments. Two of the most well-known technology-based cognitive assessment batteries were developed in the late 1980s and early 1990s using touchscreen technology. In the UK, Sahakian and colleagues published a series of papers between 1988 and 1994 (Downes *et al.* 1989; Morris *et al.* 1988; Robbins *et al.* 1994; Sahakian *et al.* 1988) describing various tasks that collectively became the Cambridge Neuropsychological Test Automated Battery (CANTAB). In France, Ritchie and collaborators produced the Examen Cognitif par Ordinateur (ECO), which was published in 1993 (Ritchie *et al.* 1993) to perform similar functions. In 2009, the Clinical Dementia Rating (CDR; Hughes *et al.* 1982), a scale commonly used by physicians for rating dementia severity, was translated and validated for use on a personal digital assistant (PDA; Galvin *et al.* 2009). Unsurprisingly, the advent of smartphones, and tablets which also use touchscreens, has further opened up opportunities for new mobile assessments such as those used to diagnose dementia. Amongst others, Weir and colleagues (2014) developed an app to diagnose dementia in a clinical setting, and Onoda and colleagues (2013) created an app for population-level screening.

Technological assessment has also extended to completion of everyday activities. Allain and colleagues (2014) asked people with AD to make a virtual cup of coffee using a virtual reality coffee machine and found that their performance on the virtual task predicted how well they carried out the task in the physical world and also how caregivers rated their abilities in completing daily tasks. Around the same time König and colleagues (2015a) tested a lab-based automated video monitoring system to assess autonomy in activities of daily living and proposed that it has potential for future home-based assessment. Assessment of people's needs for technology is examined in more detail in Chapter 2.

Cognitive rehabilitation

The potential of technology to deliver rehabilitation of cognitive functions has also long been recognised. In 1994 McConatha, McConatha and Dermigny (1994) reported an early study using an interactive computer program with older adults in long-term care (see Example 1.1).

Example 1.1 The GREET project

The GREET (Geriatric Rehabilitation Electronic Education and Training) project commenced in September 1990 to examine the potential of interactive computer training on the lives of residents in long-term care. Fourteen older adults aged between 59 and 89 years were recruited to participate, including several who were living with dementia. The study used Prodigy™, an existing online service marketed by IBM and Sears, Roebuck and Co. Prodigy™ provided a range of features including email, games, bulletin boards and an encyclopedia plus other educational and leisure resources. The GREET project ran for six months, which included training staff members at the participating long-term care units to deliver the computer intervention. Participants were trained in pairs for a minimum of three 45-minute sessions per week for two weeks, amounting to five hours of training. The study examined the impact on activities of daily living, mood and cognition and found benefits on all three. All of the participants used email, 93 per cent used games and puzzles, 85 per cent consulted consumer reports and 57 per cent checked stock market reports, while 85 per cent accessed educational materials and 78 per cent used bulletin boards. One participant reported, 'I had no idea that there was such a wide world out there. I was able to "talk" to junior high school students, share my old recipes and find out what the cheapest VCR was without leaving the building.

I also gave some advice to Lisa about her trip to Europe. This is the first time in six years I've really felt useful' (McConatha *et al.* 1994, p.555).

This pioneering work was followed by several studies, including those by Hofmann and colleagues (1996) who trained ten people with mild to moderate AD on an everyday task of individual importance, using an interactive computer program. They reported that after three weeks training, participants required less help and eight out of ten made fewer mistakes on the task. In 1999, Schreiber *et al.* trained people with dementia in real-life household tasks using MultiTask, a commercially available software. Schreiber and colleagues created an interactive, four-stage, memory training program containing pictures from graphic libraries to target immediate and delayed recall of routes and objects. Over two weeks participants received five weekly 30-minute-long treatment sessions. The goal was to train real-life household tasks in a virtual, but familiar, 3D apartment (e.g. locating objects in a room, or the route to a room within an apartment).

More recently in Hong Kong, Lee and colleagues (2013) demonstrated that a computer-based intervention developed on principles of errorless learning was as successful for people with mild to moderate dementia as the same intervention delivered by a therapist. Being able to deliver interventions remotely or online offers great possibilities to maximise the skills of therapists when one-to-one sessions are not possible. In their European project, Manera and colleagues (2015) conducted a pilot study of 'Kitchen and Cooking', a serious game developed for older adults with cognitive impairment, with 21 participants, and demonstrated that a four-week training period using the game improved concentration, but there was no investigation of transference to actual cooking tasks. Further, García-Betances and colleagues (2015) provided design criteria and strategies for the use of VR for cognitive training in dementia.

Monitoring

Technology in various forms has also been used to monitor people with dementia both at home and outside during various activities. Much of this monitoring has arisen in response to worries about the safety and security of people with dementia, for instance during activities such as cooking (Orpwood *et al.* 2008) or when leaving home unaccompanied (Sposaro, Danielson and Tyson 2010). Traditionally, such monitoring has been developed in response to concerns of families or care services rather than people living with dementia, raising many ethical issues about consent and doing things *to* people with dementia (Astell 2006). For example, the application of electronic tagging and Global Positioning Systems (GPS) as responses to people with dementia going out unaccompanied has been one of the most controversial uses of technology in dementia (Landau and Werner 2012). In 1998, McShane and colleagues examined the feasibility of electronic tracking devices through a telephone survey with 99 carers and field testing with 24 people with dementia. They concluded from the survey that 7 per cent of people with dementia in their study would have benefitted from a tracking device but identified major barriers to their use, including people with dementia not recognising the risk of getting lost and not using the device consistently. Subsequently, Hughes and Louw (2002) argued that while surveillance technology (such as tagging, which permits a third party to monitor an individual) might address the concerns of caregivers, this use of technology could dehumanise individuals with dementia by restricting their liberty and failing to take account of their views. In contrast, Bail in 2003 argued that electronic tagging offered freedom to people with dementia and provided a preferable alternative to physical restraints and locked doors. More recently smart devices that have built-in GPS, maps and accelerometers have opened up opportunities for more collaborative approaches to supporting people with dementia to continue going out alone, such as the Happy Walker project discussed in Chapter 5. Ethical issues relating to technology for dementia are explored in more depth in Chapter 3.

Everyday activities

Supporting people with dementia to continue everyday activities has been another popular focus of technology research for many years. This includes prompting in the environment to support people through the steps of a task. Several studies have investigated and elaborated COACH (Mihailidis, Barbenel and Fernie 2004), a system for supporting people in long-term care through hand-washing, using an overhead camera and sensors to detect their progress through the steps and automatically delivering voice prompting. This research was mainly carried out in the laboratory due to space requirements for setting up the system. However, current technology could make installations in long-term care environments more achievable. More recently, a feasibility study with 11 people with moderate dementia who needed assistance to complete three daily activities – drinking water, tooth brushing, upper body dressing – were able to do so 86 per cent of the time when prompted by a computer (Bewernitz *et al.* 2009). Similarly, a specially created electronic organiser tested by two people with AD successfully facilitated their daily activities (Imbeault *et al.* 2014). While the majority of such studies mentioned above are pilot or feasibility investigations with small numbers of participants, one of the largest studies of technology in the home has been taking place in Oregon (United States) since 2004. Researchers at the Oregon Centre for Aging and Technology (ORCATECH) have equipped almost 500 homes with an in-home monitoring system for sleep, gait, mobility, activity patterns, medication adherence and computer use (Lyons *et al.* 2015). They are developing algorithms to detect changes in ability and performance that may indicate significant decline and initiate interventions.

Smart homes

Delivering interventions to people with dementia directly where they live in response to changes detected in the surroundings has been another popular focus of technology research. In 2018 devices to make our homes smart are becoming increasingly popular. However, this sort of sensing and monitoring technology has been used in research in people's living environments for a number of years (see Example 1.2).

Example 1.2 Gloucester Smart House and Deptford Smart Apartment

Researchers in Bath have investigated the use of technology to anticipate the needs of people with dementia by creating first the Gloucester Smart House (Orpwood *et al.* 2004) and then a smart apartment in Deptford, London (Orpwood *et al.* 2008).

Both environments contained 'high-' and 'low-tech' features to provide a supportive and navigable environment for people with dementia. The Gloucester Smart House included monitors for the bath and cooker and a nightlight that automatically came on when a person got out of bed at night, a locator to help people find items mislaid around the house (e.g. keys) and a wall-mounted message board that could be customised to display verbal or visual messages (such as 'time for your tablets'). The assistive-living smart apartment which followed included sensors (including bed occupancy, light switches and smoke alarm), support devices (including lighting, tap control, messaging system), and speakers in each room for voice prompting, and was linked to the building's care alarm system. This apartment was evaluated by an 82-year-old man with notable cognitive impairment (a score of 10/30 on the Mini-Mental State Examination when he entered the apartment). In the four weeks before the assistive devices were activated, the sensors logged that the gentleman had an average of 3.5 hours sleep per night, often getting up during the night and then moving around the apartment. These baseline data were used to tailor a voice prompt to be delivered if he got up and was out of bed for more than 20 minutes. In the four weeks after the system was switched on his average sleep increased by more than 50 per cent to 5.4 hours. Interestingly he also regained urinary continence, which may have resulted from the prompting regarding using the toilet (Orpwood *et al.* 2008). He lived alone in the apartment for 12 months before he became physically unwell and went into hospital.

Many subsequent pilot and feasibility studies have been undertaken, particularly by engineering and computer-science researchers across the world, addressing the technical challenges of smart housing (Amiribesheli and Bouchachia 2017; Lotfi *et al.* 2012; Martin *et al.* 2007). With smart home technology becoming more widely available for anyone to use, there is huge potential for this technology to empower individuals with dementia to maintain independence and autonomy in addition to providing vital information about how people live with dementia in their own homes.

Communication

Technology-based support for communication and social interaction has also long been a focus of investigation. In 2015, Ekström, Ferm and Samuelsson reported the positive impact of a personalised intervention delivered on a tablet computer on the communication of a woman with young-onset dementia. This individualised approach was based on Computer Interactive Reminiscing and Conversation Aid (CIRCA; Alm *et al.* 2004), a touchscreen-based interactive, multimedia conversation support developed in partnership with people with dementia and caregivers. Work developing CIRCA commenced in 2001 and since that time it has been shown to provide opportunities for people with dementia to make choices and engage as an equal partner in a one-to-one conversation with a caregiver (Astell *et al.* 2008). Running successful CIRCA sessions improves staff feelings of competence as caregivers and they see people with dementia in a new light, encouraging them to re-evaluate their perceptions and expectations of their interactions with people with dementia (Astell *et al.* 2009). CIRCA also provides opportunities for enhanced wellbeing, for both staff members and people with dementia, through improved positive relations (Astell *et al.* 2010). Further exploration has demonstrated that CIRCA can accommodate diversity and elicit different perspectives from across cultural groups by acting as a third party in a conversation (Purves *et al.* 2015). This has led to the creation a web-based version of CIRCA that can be populated with contents from different cultures and languages that is currently being tested in Sweden, the Netherlands and Spain. This has been validated in a multi-session group-based activity for delivering cognitive stimulation to people living with dementia (Astell *et al.* 2018b).

Fun and games

The final area to mention is the use of technology to support people with dementia to engage with and enjoy leisure activities. Following the success of CIRCA, the same team started working in 2004 with people who have dementia to develop interactive touchscreen games. More than 30 activities were developed and evaluated, resulting in a set of basic activities that people with dementia could play independently (Astell *et al.* 2014a). This work has rapidly expanded with the advent and widescale availability of touchscreen devices and is further explored in Chapter 7, while the use of an existing gaming system by people with dementia is described below.

Caregiving

For formal caregivers, a range of web-based training interventions have been developed. The CARES programme developed for nursing assistants was shown to improve retention of new information and skills and reduce stress relating to caregiving (Hobday *et al.* 2010). Technology has also been applied to creating integrated care packages for people with dementia, such as the intervention management system developed by Eichler and colleagues to suggest recommendations to GPs (Eichler *et al.* 2016).

An early study exploring the potential of digital support for family caregivers, conducted by Brennan, Moore and Smyth in 1991, found that nursing support could be delivered remotely to enhance care at home. More recently Boots and colleagues (2014) found that interacting with an online coach or other caregivers could benefit informal caregivers and support their own mental health and wellbeing, but systematic evaluation of Internet-based training and support is lacking. Regarding the use of technology to assist with caregiving, a survey of 72 family caregivers identified that devices they perceived as having high usefulness were familiar, intuitive, easy to use, simplified activities and prevented accidents, with safety often given priority over the privacy and autonomy of their relatives with dementia (Mao *et al.* 2015). Considering the early start of this work, the results of a 2018 review of mobile apps targeting caregivers by Grossman, Zak and Zelinski (2018) are rather surprising. In October 2017 they identified only 44 apps out of approximately 200,000 healthcare apps in Google Play and iTunes. Analysis of these apps found they focused on five main areas: information and resources, practical problem solving, family communication, interaction with care-recipient and caregiver support. Few apps were comprehensive, i.e. addressing more than one area. The range and availability of technologies to support informal caregivers is addressed more fully in Chapter 8 and formal caregivers in organisations in Chapter 9.

Types of technology for dementia

The list of research areas covered here is illustrative rather than exhaustive, and many more examples are to be found in the chapters of this book. Corresponding to the large range of areas tackled, a similarly large range of technologies has been explored as solutions and supports for people living with dementia, their families and friends, and health and social care providers. These include existing mainstream devices such as personal computers, mobile telephones, tablet computers, digital games systems, wearables and environmental sensors. Some of these have been applied as is, for example the Xbox Kinect motion-based game system (Dove and Astell 2017a; see Case study 1.1) and touchscreen tablet computers (Astell *et al.* 2016), while others have been adapted for dementia, including a reminding system developed for a mobile phone (Nugent *et al.* 2008). The range of functions include software applications, web-based services, and devices that people can wear or attach to their clothing. A number of technologies such as CIRCA (Alm *et al.* 2004), a touchscreen-based support for art therapy (Leuty *et al.* 2013) and another to promote musical creativity (Riley, Alm and Newell 2009) have been specially created for people living with dementia. The potential of robots has also attracted attention, with multiple projects exploring both commercially available ones, such as 'Giraff' (Kristoffersson, Coradeschi and Loutfi 2013), and developing new ones, such as 'Brian' (McColl, Chan and Nejat 2012), specifically for dementia (see below).

Motion-based technology

Many care settings offer group activities as these place fewer demands on staff resources. However, it can be challenging to identify group activities that are engaging and accessible for people living with dementia. Motion-based technologies (MBT; e.g. Nintendo Wii, Xbox Kinect) can be used in both group and individual settings to offer engaging activities to people with dementia (Dove and Astell 2017a). Furthermore, the movements required to interact with this type of technology are intuitive ones that resemble everyday actions (e.g. reaching out to the side), resulting in an accessible interaction for people with a wide range of abilities.

While the first motion-based, hand-held game controller was created in 1981, motion-based technologies have only recently begun to emerge in dementia research and care. For example, a comprehensive review of the literature of the use of motion-based technology by people with dementia or mild cognitive impairment (MCI) in 2017 identified only 31 studies, all of which were published in the previous ten years (i.e. 2007–2017; Dove and Astell 2017c). Of these 31 studies, 26 utilised the Nintendo Wii or Microsoft Xbox Kinect, suggesting that the release of these technologies in 2006 and 2010 respectively inspired the use of motion-based technologies for people living with dementia.

Case study 1.1 The Kinect project

Motion-based technologies provide opportunities to bring cognitive, physical and leisure activities into care contexts such as adult day programmes, assisted living facilities and long-term care homes (Dove and Astell 2017c). We recently tested a 20-session Xbox Kinect bowling program in an adult day programme as a regularly scheduled group activity to examine how best to introduce these gaming activities (Dove and Astell 2017a). Gameplay sessions lasting approximately one hour each took place twice a week for ten weeks (see Figure 1.1). Sessions were facilitated by a member of the research team ('the trainer'), who introduced, taught and supported participants to use the technology. We applied training techniques identified in the literature (Dove and Astell 2017c) and a previous study observing people with dementia playing Xbox Kinect games (Dove and Astell 2017b). We recorded the sessions using two video cameras, which were positioned at the front and back of the room to capture (1) the actions of the trainer and the participants, (2) gameplay outcomes (e.g. bowling a strike), (3) facial expressions and (4) the group dynamic.

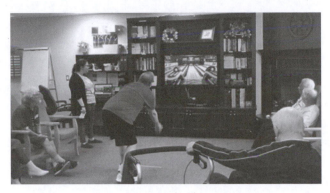

Figure 1.1 Kinect bowling group

Results demonstrate that appropriate training and support enable people with dementia to learn to play MBT games independently. Techniques such as task breakdown plus verbal, gestural and physical assistance prompts were useful in teaching people with dementia to use MBT. This was evident through a reduced need for trainer instruction, increased ability to play independently and shorter duration of turns (Dove, Cotnam and Astell 2017). These results highlight the learning capabilities of people with dementia, particularly in relation to meaningful activities and skills (Kessels *et al.* 2013), which challenge stigma and negative stereotypes regarding the abilities of people with dementia.

As we observed previously, participants engaged with the technology both independently and collaboratively. For example, while each participant played the turn individually, other members of the group supported them by cheering, clapping, laughing and offering encouraging comments. Additionally, participants frequently engaged in friendly teasing and mild competition. For example:

'Yeah, you guys gotta get it!' (Participant 02)

'Come on [participant name], you're supposed to show us how it's done!' (Participant 08)

'Show off!' (Participant 06)

Furthermore, participants reported enjoying the activity, suggesting that this type of programme can be used as a regular group activity for people with dementia. For example:

'I always look forward to Mondays and Fridays, because I know it's bowling day.' (Participant 08)

'This is fun, I like this game.' (Participant 07)

In summary, our results suggest that using MBTs, such as the Xbox Kinect, can deliver positive benefits for people with dementia. Based on these results we have implemented Kinect bowling groups in four day programmes and produced a paper containing guidelines for MBT system development and use for people with dementia (Astell, Czarnuch and Dove 2018a).

Robots

Research into robotics generally has gathered pace over recent years. In healthcare for older adults, efforts fall into several areas including robots as direct caregivers, robots as assistants, robots as companions and robots as facilitators of social interaction. Coughlin (2015) suggested that robots could provide a solution to the predicted 'caregiver crisis' and potentially reduce the sky-rocketing costs of long-term care (approximately $219.9 billion in the US in 2012) and $522 billion per annum of informal, unpaid caregiving provided by family or friends of the care recipient. The possibility of robot carers has also been investigated for a number of years (see Example 1.3).

Example 1.3 NurseBot

In the 1990s a team from Carnegie Mellon University in the United States established the NurseBot project to develop a robot to support older adults with mild cognitive and physical impairments as well as support nurses in their daily activities. Building on their previous work with 'Flo' (after Florence Nightingale), 'Pearl' (aka NurseBot) was created to address a number of challenges in creating an assistant or companion to replace a human caregiver. These included how humanoid the robot should look, whether the robot should display emotion, and how it might interact with people, e.g. through speech or through text or both (Roy *et al.* 2000). In 2003 the team reported that their mobile robotic assistant autonomously provided prompts and guidance to older adults during trials in an assisted living facility (Pineau *et al.* 2003) and in 2005 Pearl was a finalist in the INDEX awards (INDEX 2011). What became of Pearl after that is unknown. However, the pursuit of a robot caregiver has continued, with examples including the RoboBear from Japan and Giraffplus from Europe.

More recently telepresence robots or robots for social interaction have been the focus of much research in dementia. Telepresence robots are basically a video conferencing system controlled by a remote user, i.e. rather than appearing on a fixed desktop monitor or screen, the person speaking can move the robot around the environment from their own location. Currently a range of telepresence robots are available to purchase, including Giraff, Anybots, Beampro®, VGo, Double Robotics and MantaroBot (Kristoffersson *et al.* 2013). Of these, Giraff has been developed and used in a number of European research projects, such as Giraffplus (Coradeschi *et al.* 2013), focused on supporting older adults at home by combining the robot with a network of sensors.

Another support robot is Brian (McColl *et al.* 2012), a humanoid robot developed to support people living with dementia in long-term care facilities at mealtimes. Brian was created to address the need for one-to-one support to encourage people with dementia to eat through prompting, which places large demands on care staff. Sensors on crockery were used for activity recognition, with emotion recognised through a front webcam and facial recognition software. In a feasibility study Brian was able to learn a selection of assistive behaviours appropriate to the meal and personalise interactions based on the individual's response to the task and their emotional response while interacting. The same researchers have also been involved in the development of Casper (Bovbel and Nejat 2014), a prototype robot to prompt people through the steps of meal preparation, and Tangy (Louie *et al.* 2015), a non-humanoid robot to support bingo in care homes.

Summary

Although research into technology for dementia has been under way for many years, it has been at a far smaller scale than biomedical research, in terms of funding and number of projects. This is largely because the focus of research funding has been on trying to find a cure, with less emphasis, until recently, on supporting people who have dementia to live as well as possible. In this respect, technology research has tackled a much wider range of issues than biomedical research and is more comparable with efforts made in psychosocial research. Technological studies pose a number of novel ethical questions and challenges relating to privacy, responsibility, data security, autonomy, freedom and control. Technology studies also raise issues about access to and availability of apps, devices and services. By focusing on challenges relating to living with dementia, technology studies go beyond the purely medical symptoms, raising further questions about who should provide the new devices and systems, i.e. are they health-related or not?

Take-home points

* Research into technology for dementia has been under way for many years.

* Technology research has been funded to a much smaller extent than biomedical research which has limited the amount and speed of progress.

* Currently available commercial technologies contain many functions that can support people to live well with dementia, but need to be in people's hands as early as possible.

* Family caregivers can benefit from technology including information, resources, problem solving, education, peer support and communication.

* Organisations can utilise technology to support their workforce, clients and their families across all aspects of their services.

Acknowledgements

We are grateful to the people living with dementia, their families and caregivers who have shared their experiences and contributed to the development of the ideas expressed in this chapter, with a special mention for our friends at Oshawa Senior Citizen's Centres (OSCC), Oshawa, Canada. We also acknowledge funding for our research from the Canadian Consortium on Neurodegeneration and Aging (CCNA) and AGE-WELL, Canada's ageing and technology network.

Chapter 2

Assessing the Needs of People with Dementia for Technology

Professor Louise Nygård, *Professor of Occupational Therapy, Department of Neurobiology, Care Sciences and Society, Division of Occupational Therapy, Karolinska Institute, Sweden*

Dr Camilla Malinowsky, *Assistant Professor, Department of Neurobiology, Care Sciences and Society, Division of Occupational Therapy, Karolinska Institute, Sweden*

Dr Lena Rosenberg, *Assistant Professor, Department of Neurobiology, Care Sciences and Society, Division of Occupational Therapy, Karolinska Institute, Sweden*

Introduction

In this chapter, we approach needs from a pragmatic point of view. This means that we focus on needs related to managing daily life, rather than generic human needs (such as those proposed by, for example, Maslow in 1943). Many studies have explored the needs commonly experienced by people living with dementia and care partners, suggesting that information and support with regard to symptoms, safety, belongingness, social contacts and relationships, and being useful and engaged in meaningful activities, are priorities (Pini *et al.* 2018; Schölzel-Dorenbos, Meeuwsen and Olde Rikkert 2010). Taking the point of departure in management of daily life, the need to be engaged in activities that are perceived as meaningful and fulfilling by the individual, embracing doing as well as being and becoming (Wilcock 1999), is in the forefront in this chapter. This generic need also goes for people living with dementia – although their possibilities to fulfil the need of activity engagement will be influenced by the consequences of the disease. With this view, needs are not necessarily emanating from common disease symptoms such as memory deficits and deteriorating orientation to time, space and identity, but rather to the experienced consequences of these symptoms as they come to the fore in each individual's specific everyday life situation and context.

How to identify needs of people with dementia (for technology): Where do we start?

When considering how to identify needs of people with dementia we must ask ourselves: What is a need? Who determines a person's need? A need is not the same as a symptom, an impairment or an obvious problem. A person who, for example, has difficulty remembering appointments does not necessarily experience a need to remember appointments. Hence, a symptom of memory decline or an identified difficulty in daily life activities does not necessarily translate into an experienced need to manage these difficulties. However, in this example, people around the person who does not remember appointments will be likely to experience that there is a need to find a solution – but who then has the need?

Widening the view: Power relationships and autonomy

When it comes to people living with dementia, we have to broaden the perspective from a purely individualised view to including, for example, both parts of a couple where one is diagnosed with dementia, or other persons that are close to the one with dementia. This is not to say that the person with dementia is unable to express needs, but rather to acknowledge that the consequences of dementia typically involve also those close to the person. Yet, we also have to be very attentive to the needs that are expressed by the person living with dementia, because the person may be less likely to eloquently and explicitly explain what is needed and why, while others around the person may be more likely to make their voices heard (Rosenberg and Nygård 2012). It is also important to pay attention to this power relationship when we try to understand the needs of people with dementia and their care partners or significant others and the potential of technology as solutions, as aspects of meaning might overrule pragmatic concerns (Nygård 2008). The possibility to express one's needs is also closely related to autonomy, i.e. self-rule. To not restrain the autonomy of the person with dementia requires an activity- and problem-oriented approach towards the needs expressed by the person.

As healthcare professionals, we often tend to think along very function-oriented lines, focusing on solving problems related to functioning in daily life but not always acknowledging the importance of who the person living with dementia is, or wants to be, how he or she identifies him or herself, or wants to be perceived by others. Moreover, we are first and foremost trained to aim for solving problems that interfere with people's independence; for example, if the person could manage cooking, that would ease the responsibilities and costs of home helpers or burden on significant others. Hence, we are likely to assume that difficulties in cooking convey a need for solutions – without always considering if that is important for the person. It might, for example, be the case that a person's image of self rests strongly on other features, suggesting that other activities and roles than the ones healthcare professionals are traditionally trained to monitor are most important and result in needs for support. In other words, the activities we engage in contribute to who we are; our actions create us and show our belonging, who we are and who we want to be (Wilcock 1999). This, of course, is also the case for people who live with dementia, and these aspects will inevitably influence the needs they experience (Greenhalgh *et al.* 2013; Nygård, Borell and Gustavsson 1995).

To be attentive to the person with dementia and gain knowledge about the activities and roles that are meaningful and important for him or her will enable us to support the person to continue living the life that he or she wishes to live. This can also be regarded as retained self-rule; that is, autonomy.

One especially pronounced need, emphasised by both people living with dementia and those close to them, is the need for social engagement (Pini *et al.* 2018; Schölzel-Dorenbos *et al.* 2010). Social life and social activities, especially those outside home, are often increasingly compromised as dementia evolves, and withdrawal is for some the ultimate choice when no other solutions are found.

Needs may be mutable

Another particularly important aspect to pay attention to is the unstable nature of dementia; as it is a progressive disease this means that needs might change, or come in different shapes as time passes, as the life situation changes, or the disease progresses. This implies that it is important to follow the persons with dementia and their significant others over time to capture needs that emerge over time. In a study where we examined the lived experiences of learning and maintaining knowledge relating to technology among people with dementia, we learnt that not only changes in the person's abilities but also the ever-changing nature of technology artefacts and services influenced whether the person with dementia could continue to use certain technologies or not (Rosenberg and Nygård 2017). Another example was provided by people with dementia who took part in a study aimed at developing an easy-to-use video-telephone for people with dementia. Participants emphasised how important it would be to develop the telephone in different versions; a small portable one to be used while still mobile and fairly competent, and a large stationary one to be used when the disease requires the person to stay put and rely on a habitual environment (Boman, Nygård and Rosenberg 2014b).

Meanings

Just as everyday activities carry meanings for all of us, technologies are also given meanings; they are by no means neutral to us, but loaded with individual as well as shared meanings. On the one hand, for some people, technology can add status if it is regarded a symbol of, for example, being up to date, or being the same as everybody else, as might be the case for digital goods such as iPads (Greenhalgh *et al.* 2013; Nygård 2008; Rosenberg, Kottorp and Nygård 2012). On the other hand, technology can also be perceived as stigmatising if the person feels that it might expose him or her as different or divergent from others (Greenhalgh *et al.* 2013). This showed clearly in two studies where people living with Alzheimer's disease needed support from devices to help them manage time and everyday life. In both studies, participants rejected using memory aids with audio reminders although they acknowledged needing these reminders; the risk of the aid exposing them as different if it started to give instructions in public situations was experienced as stigmatising (Nygård and Johansson 2001; Rosenberg and Nygård 2012). The risk of stigmatisation by technology has also been expressed by significant others of people living with dementia. For example, non-stigmatising appearance of the technology was found to be a prerequisite for acceptance and successful incorporation of technology in one study involving family care partners (Rosenberg *et al.* 2012); some technologies were suggested to be perceived as stigmatising the user simply because they were associated with old age.

Trying out and exploring possibilities

It might also be difficult to articulate and define what a person needs, even if a broad area such as timing is identified as a challenge that the person explicitly wishes to maintain mastery of (Nygård and Johansson 2001). In the earlier-mentioned case study (Rosenberg and Nygård 2012), the need of a person who lived by herself with help from home care was formulated as a need to keep appointments and to know beforehand when home helpers would come to bring the laundry and take her grocery shopping. This prospective time management issue was identified as most urgent by herself, as well as by those close to her. Different devices were tried out with the goal to support her mastery of time. However, over time it became obvious that from her view, the most important thing regarding time was to recall the things that *had* happened (e.g. knowing what day she had washed her hair), i.e. looking back, even though this was not a need that she, or anyone else, had been able to articulate beforehand. This exemplifies that it might be difficult to know the potential of the technology before having tried it in everyday life. It is easier to identify what specific needs the technology is expected to target, for example, remembering when to take medication, or supporting orientation in space, than understanding precisely *how* to utilise a device to support a particular person's everyday life. Therefore, this must be tried out in each individual case, acknowledging that there might be individual needs that had not been given conscious attention or that could not be explicitly expressed before someone recognised and tried to solve an issue.

In the example above, the people close to the woman with dementia had their own ideas about her needs. Her daughter prioritised using the time device to help her mother to keep track of what was to come (e.g. reminders of healthcare appointments), and the home helpers prioritised using the device to remind her of activities that they were responsible for (e.g. preparing meals). Soon her newly discovered need to keep track of what had happened was being ignored. This exemplifies what might happen when there are conflicting ideas about what is the most relevant and important aspect of an identified need (e.g. time management as reminders for future events, or support to remember past events) – especially when the person needs support to set and make use of the device. When such a conflict emerges, there is an eminent risk that the voice of the person with dementia will be the weakest, as power relationships are seldom equal when dementia is present (Rosenberg and Nygård 2012).

Two points of departure

We can illustrate the reasoning above on 'How can we identify a need?' by using two different starting points: (1) knowing a technology and this technology's potential, or (2) identifying what is important for the person in terms of doing, being and becoming: that is, from the person's needs.

Departing from the technology's potential

An activity- and problem-oriented approach, focusing on the priorities of the person living with dementia and those close to the person, will probably be the most useful point of departure when trying to identify needs and the solutions to these, but it is still a fact that new technologies and their functions might be discovered to have potential areas of use that we did not think of when being introduced to them. Often, technological development emanates from constructive and creative ideas about how adding or adjusting features of a technology might open up new usage situations. For example, apps for smartphones are developed to guide a person's wayfinding – and indeed apps are today developed and used for many purposes taking this point of departure. It has been suggested that touchscreens are perceived as intuitive and attractive by people with dementia (Boman *et al.* 2014a; Joddrell 2017), and the development of apps for smartphones and tablets for different purposes is ever so lively. However, we do not know to what extent the potential of apps in smartphones and tablets will match the needs of people living with dementia when it comes to their priorities and challenges in daily life activities. We will come back to this a little later.

Knowing brings creative possibilities

No doubt, the creativity of people living with dementia and their significant others should not be underestimated; it is indeed possible that they come up with their own ways of using technology, given that it matches their needs. Also, people with dementia bring their own ideas about how to bring technological objects and functions into play. For example, in one study a man with Alzheimer's disease experienced a very uncomfortable confusion about the direction of time. From his own initiative, he had started to use the digital time shown on teletext to keep a sense of existential order, and sitting down just watching this for a while made him feel more at ease (Nygård 2008). This is just one example of many that show that people living with dementia might also find their own and novel solutions – with or without technology. These inventive solutions may be further supported by people close to the individual if they seem to work well and fulfil a need of the person living with dementia.

Similarly, getting to know that certain technologies exist that have the potential to support people's daily life activities and solve problems can inspire care partners and persons living with dementia to try out how these might be used in individual cases. The technology is then applied by matching its potential to common, known or anticipated problems, or by focusing on compensation for an existing impairment. Family care partners in research studies have expressed how important it might be to know of available technologies, sometimes in preparation for problems that might appear later on (Nygård 2009; Rosenberg *et al.* 2012). For example, stove timers have been regularly installed in people's homes in some Swedish municipalities for people with impaired memory (Nygård, Starkhammar and Lilja 2008). There are also examples showing that learning how to use a technology for the utilisation of one feature (e.g. time information) might be decisive for later on accepting and incorporating yet another function (e.g. reminders) when new needs eventually appear (Boman *et al.* 2014b).

The risk of mismatches

We also want to share one example of how focus on a technology, and the influence of what is possible to do, can cause a mismatch with expressed wishes or needs if these are not attended to. As mentioned earlier, stove timers have in some Swedish municipalities been installed without costs for the inhabitant if a professional certifies that use of the stove implies a risk due to memory deficits. As safety is regarded as a primary issue, it is likely to be prioritised and interpreted as a need in a 'one size fits all' approach where health and social service staff have little time to listen to other needs. In our research data, there were multiple examples of older adults with memory issues who had received a stove timer because there were routines for prescribing stove timers, and staff felt that they by doing that, they at least could do something – even if the timer did not match any individual needs of their clients (Nygård 2009). This meant that to some extent they solved the problem of risk of fire, which of course is a main issue. However, the stove timer in many cases became an obstacle to maintaining activity rather than a facilitator, partly because the options for individual settings were not used or adjusted once the timing device had been installed: an example of the focus being set on the technology rather than the individual users' needs (Nygård *et al.* 2008; Starkhammar and Nygård 2008). Because of this, the technology did not support the person to maintain his or her activities and wellbeing in the long run (Nygård 2009).

Departing from the person's needs

The other point of departure, which we propose should always be taken into consideration, is 'What is important for the person to do in everyday life, and why?' Then the need identification would, for example, focus on how to maintain continued engagement in a particular activity, or how to find other, alternative activities or solutions to specific issues. This could mean solving a problem in the performance of an activity, or adapting how an activity is performed, keeping the need that the activity fulfils for the individual in mind. For example, spending time outside home by going to the grocery store might be related to a variety of needs beside buying groceries, e.g. getting exercise, meeting people, breathing fresh air (Brorsson *et al.* 2011). This also exemplifies that each activity may be given a variety of meanings. If only the need to get groceries is acknowledged, then the solution could be to do shopping online or to have somebody to bring the groceries, which would risk leaving many other needs unattended. By adding a new component (e.g. technology) in the performance of an activity, we might also profoundly change the meaning of the activity for the person, thus ruling out technology as a solution or equally finding that technology actually adds value (Lindqvist, Larsson and Borell 2015).

Attending to the priorities of people with dementia

What types of everyday activities do people with mild cognitive impairment or early-stage dementia want to maintain mastery of, and why? This might seem to be an odd question to ask – why should their wishes be different from any others'? However, it is well known that there are many different ideas about what older adults, and especially people living with dementia, should or should not do. For example, safety is usually an issue both for persons living with dementia (Sandberg *et al.* 2017) and, sometimes even more so, for their care partners (Greenhalgh *et al.* 2013; Rosenberg *et al.* 2012). A literature review (Lindqvist *et al.* 2016) found that very few studies had raised the question about the priorities of people living with dementia. In the review, they found four types of activities that were most important for these persons. These were activities that (1) conveyed social values and wellbeing (e.g. engaging in baking, socialising, going for a walk), (2) supported significant roles (e.g. going to the cinema conveyed that the person was an active part of society), (3) diminished negative influence on other people (e.g. managing regular meals reduced the worries of family) and (4) increased health and safety (e.g. mastering of leaving home in a controlled manner, or paying in a safe way in shops).

These findings in part confirm that the needs of people living with dementia are related to social life, relationships and safety, as identified by Schölzel-Dorenbos *et al.* (2010), but the new findings also showed how doing and being were intertwined, for example in maintaining roles through engagement in valued activities. While the four areas found in the literature review might present a starting point when checking for needs of support through or in technology use, the study's findings point to another important issue: managing some activities were in fact a 'prerequisite for accomplishing other activities, that is, they had to precede other desired activities, which was interpreted as a form of dependency between the activities' (Lindqvist *et al.* 2016, p.403). This showed that some of the challenging activities were not always desired for their own sake, but for enabling another more valued activity. Many challenges were related to the requirement of ability to use technology. Again, this exemplifies the complexity of understanding what needs people living with dementia might have, and also the multifaceted nature of technology as a challenge as well as a potential solution.

Enjoyment and relaxation

Lindqvist and colleagues' review (2016) also points to the need of activity engagement for wellbeing, and reminds us of the fact that enjoyment is an important aspect of wellbeing. The importance of relaxation and enjoyment through entertainment has received increased attention in research related to dementia. This is illustrated, for example, in the developing field of gaming that incorporates accessibility settings designed specifically for people living with dementia (Joddrell 2017). Similarly, the development of communication technologies to facilitate social engagement with family and friends for older adults living with dementia has received much attention (Boman *et al.* 2014a). There are also shared ideas in society about morality and technology use; while using technology for playing games might be perceived as healthy training for older adults, watching television is often regarded as a passive and less healthy activity. For example, Rosenberg *et al.* (2012) found that some family care partners even hoped for a slower course of the cognitive decline for a person with dementia who kept on using technologies that required the use of codes and spent much time at the computer, assuming that this meant healthy brain training. They concluded: 'Generally, engaging in challenging tasks by using technology was seen by the participants as an exercise opportunity in everyday life' (p.517). In contrast, spending time watching television was seen by the care partners as creating passivity and thus being less health promoting.

Interestingly, another study in a Swedish group living facility for people with dementia found that watching commercials was an especially favourite activity according to residents, as these featured short, vivid and engaging narratives, and the viewers were actively engaged in an enjoyable activity (Östlund 2010). This again shows how activities, as well as technologies, are given different values, which will also influence what needs are recognised and what steps are taken to fulfil the needs. No doubt there is a large potential for technology to fill needs related to both cognitive stimulation and enjoyment – if used with conscious awareness of the person's expressions of what is enjoyable or what he or she wish to do, rather than the social environment's priorities and views on 'what is best' for the individual.

The process of asking questions

Inevitably, the mere availability of a smart technology still leads us to queries such as: What needs can be met by this technology and how, when, for whom? But we still face the question: What is a need and according to whom? That question is still necessary, and provides a fundamental base in the process of asking other questions related to this topic, as elaborated on below. From both the starting points discussed above, we will end up with the same negotiations and considerations of how the technology responds to the person's priorities and needs for support; for example, a value identified by the person with dementia, a limitation or problem to solve, an activity to facilitate or just to provide pleasure, enjoyment or relaxation, with a clear idea of who sets the priority.

Suggested questions to ask

Some years ago, we developed a simple conversation tool for healthcare staff with questions to ask in the process of guiding a person with dementia and/or his or her significant others (Rosenberg and Nygård 2010). This was based on qualitative studies involving both people with dementia and their significant others. The tool suggests a set of aspects to consider in initial conversations with a person with dementia and his or her significant other around technology and everyday life, for example:

- Talk about using everyday technology, and whether there are any issues in using it, taking the point of departure in the activities that the person with dementia engages in. Focus on the technologies that are relevant in the person's everyday life (e.g. television, telephone, ATM).

- Find out if the person and/or significant other have developed their own ways to use everyday technology, or if adaptations have been made. If so, why have these adaptations been made and how do they work?

- Find out if there are any technologies that are particularly important for the self-image of the person with dementia, and for how the person wishes to be seen by others, and find out if there are any issues when using it.

- Keep in mind that there might be colliding needs and views on the situation in the person with dementia and the significant others.

Further, the tool also suggests questions to be asked when giving advice, prescribing technologies or evaluating support from technology to persons with dementia and significant others, for example:

- Before introducing the technology, make sure that the person with dementia him or herself perceives a need for the technological support, or has an interest in trying to use it.

- Make sure that the technology in question fits the unique situation of the particular person and his or her significant others. Aspects such as age, living alone or cohabiting, vocational status and familiarity with technology may all affect the outcome.

- Keep in mind that it should be possible to intuitively trace out or guess how to use the technology *in the midst of it being used*. This is important because it is likely that the person with dementia will have difficulty remembering instructions or reading user manuals.

Matching is a continuous process

When trying to identify and understand the need a person living with dementia might have for technology to facilitate daily life, and to meet this need with such a solution, we might think of the potential fit or match between the nature of the problem, the person's wishes and abilities, and the potential and requirements of the technology. For example, a person might need support to be able to spend time outdoors, in order to socialise, exercise and buy groceries. Our first solution idea might be to use an app on a smartphone, providing instructions for orientation – but does the ability of the person match the requirements of the smartphone technology and the features of the app (if a smartphone is available)? If the smartphone is new to the person, what is the possibility of him or her learning how to use it? What meanings are attached to the smartphone by the person and others, and how would these meanings influence the possibility of eventually using the technology as successful support in the particular situations?

When introducing the idea of a match between technologies and people, we want to stress that this is always a process; a match today might be a mismatch tomorrow, for many different reasons. It has been suggested that professionals should maintain an open and flexible approach towards goal setting with their clients living with dementia, as the goal of an intervention (e.g. support through technology) might be adjusted in the process of incorporating the device in the routines of everyday life. An alternative to goal setting could be to identify potential 'ends in view', reflecting the reciprocal character of ends and means (Dewey 1981), as this concept acknowledges the process of striving for a solution to a problem in a more explorative way (Rosenberg and Nygård 2012).

Assessing ability to use technology

In our earlier research, two assessment instruments capturing people's ability to use technology have been developed and validated: Everyday Technology Use Questionnaire (ETUQ; Nygård *et al.* 2012; Rosenberg, Nygård and Kottorp 2009), and Management of Everyday Technology Assessment (META; Malinowsky *et al.* 2010; Malinowsky, Nygård and Kottorp 2011). Importantly, these instruments do not assess a person's ability to perform or engage in activities, but they measure one specific aspect of that: the ability to use technology. In research with these instruments, a person's ability as technology user can be directly related to the level of challenge of more than 90 common everyday technologies. In other words, the match between a person and the technology is displayed. So far, this is only possible in research, but in the future – given the development of these tools as computer adaptive testing (CAT) – it might also be possible for clinical healthcare staff, particularly occupational therapists, to check this match while in the process of investigating a person's activity limitations and goals, including the ability to use technology (Kottorp and Nygård 2011). In clinical practice, assessments with the META can add information of the performance in the use of relevant technologies by mapping out the observed ability to perform actions important in technology use, for example choosing the correct button or command and performing steps and actions in a logical sequence (Malinowsky *et al.* 2010, 2011). These performance actions, i.e. skills, emanate from an empirical, explorative study of people living with dementia and how they used their own everyday technologies (Nygård and Starkhammar 2007). This research has also shown that some performance action skills are more challenging than others; for example, noticing information and responding adequately is demonstrated to be the most difficult skill, and identifying and selecting/separating technologies the easiest, among older adults with and without cognitive impairment or dementia. Knowledge of the level of challenge for skills needed in the use of technology can be used to guide interventions aiming to support technology use or when choosing assistive technology or setting the features of a technology (Malinowsky, Kottorp and Nygård 2013).

Usability

One key issue in many of the examples we have given in this chapter is related to the concept of usability. Usability is a concept often referred to for clarifying the match between the requirements of technology and the potentials of the user, and it is commonly defined as 'The extent to which a system, product or service can be used by specific users to achieve specified goals with effectiveness, efficiency and satisfaction in a specified context of use' (International Organization for Standardization 2018). In other words, if a person's need is to be met by utilisation of technology, the usability of the technology for that person in that situation must be adequate.

A few examples from research will illuminate the issue of usability in the context of people living with dementia. The results of our earlier research show that what is communicated through the interface of a technology is particularly crucial for its usability, as this is likely to guide the person with dementia through suitable use, whereas instructions are likely to be forgotten (Rosenberg and Nygård 2012). Findings from a study on how people with mild cognitive impairment (MCI) or dementia approached learning related to technology demonstrated how the design of the technology interacts with the user and his or her process of learning in the ways that the technology communicates with the user (Rosenberg and Nygård 2014). These examples highlight that the user interface of the technology is crucial both for learning and for usability. In a qualitative usability analysis of empirical data from participants with dementia or stroke, Lindqvist and colleagues (2015) found that the features in assistive technologies that enhanced the users' sense of control were most important for their achievement of goals; that is, for meeting their needs. The importance of trust in the technology as really 'working' has been emphasised in many studies; for example, in Greenhalgh and colleagues' study (2013) and in an evaluation of support through technology for people living with dementia (Lindqvist, Nygård and Borell 2013) where the issue of coverage and access to the Internet emerged as a key aspect for becoming a user of the support. Furthermore, other important usability features in the usability analysis were how the technology was maintained and communicated with other technology.

Possible future paths

According to Greenhalgh *et al.* (2013), successful solutions to older adults' needs often require adaptation or customisation of the technology, involving different people, including professionals, close to the one in need of support. In their study, they found that such 'bricolage' had been used in successful technology solutions; that is, pragmatic customisations where new devices or components had been adapted and/or combined with systems or materials already existing in the homes of older adults in need of assistance. Similar ideas of how everyday technologies and assistive devices could be combined were given by occupational therapists in another study; for instance, how a hearing aid could be combined with the television set and the telephone (Nygård and Rosenberg 2016). These studies underscore the importance of making sure that different technologies or technological systems, new and existing, communicate. Interestingly, Greenhalgh *et al.* (2013) found bricolage to be common when it came to everyday technologies such as computers and kitchen technologies, but rarely seen with assistive technologies. They also emphasised that in-depth understanding of the older adult's needs and relating these to existing and/or new technologies were prerequisites for successful solutions. We propose the idea of bricolage as an interesting venue for further research when it comes to using technology to support people living with dementia. This will require reconsideration of how to identify and meet these people's needs, and how to evaluate the technological support, as the matter is complex, and involves many parties in the person's context, requiring joint actions and continuous adaptations and customisations.

We also propose that it is imperative to acknowledge the complexity and organic nature of the interplay between people and technologies in real-life activities, situations and environments that cannot be controlled but often are shared, and where continuous changes will take place in all facets of the interplay. This view underscores that collaboration between many disciplines and stakeholders is needed if people with dementia are to truly benefit from technological development.

Take-home points

* Understanding the needs of a person with dementia for technology/ support requires that attention is given to the person's priorities – even if these may be less explicitly expressed than the priorities of others in the person's vicinity.

* Technologies are given meanings by people with dementia as well as by their care partners and other people and societies; such meanings matter and might change over time – an explorative and flexible approach is recommended.

* Focusing on technology's potential brings about a risk of not meeting the person's needs but can also show new creative possibilities if used with awareness and caution.

* Paying attention to the priorities of the person with dementia includes not only attending to activities that are important for independence but also activities for enjoyment, social life and relaxation.

* There are tools developed based upon empirical research that can guide healthcare professionals in asking questions and assessing people's ability to use technology.

* The complex and organic interplay between people and technologies in real-life activities, situations and environments cannot be ignored; one way to practise that perspective is to use or be inspired by the idea of bricolage.

Chapter 3

Ethical Issues in Technology for Dementia

Dr Jennifer Boger, *Assistant Professor,*
Systems Design Engineering and Schlegel Research Chair for Technology
in Independent Living, University of Waterloo, Canada

Professor Jeffrey Jutai, *Interdisciplinary School of Health Sciences,*
University of Ottawa, Canada

Dr Anne Moorhead, *Senior Lecturer in Health*
Communication, Ulster University, UK

Professor Maurice Mulvenna, *Professor of Computer Science,*
School of Computing, Ulster University, UK

Dr Raymond Bond, *Senior Lecturer in Data Analytics, Ulster University, UK*

Introduction

The pervasiveness, complexity and sophistication of technology are increasing at a phenomenal rate. While this growth is enabling technology to play a more prominent role in supporting people living with dementia and their care partners in a wide variety of ways, we encounter new situations and questions regarding how and when it should be used: Who chooses when technologies are used? Who has control over the data they collect? And how can technologies be designed to be inherently more ethical?

Governments, industry, not-for-profit organisations and society in general are starting to consider these questions. For example, the WHO Global Health Ethics team held an initial meeting at the University of Tübingen, Germany on 18 March 2017 to discuss the development of a framework to address ethical issues related to ageing and health, including ethical guidance for healthcare rationing, assistive devices and health environments. The European Dementia Ethics Network, founded in 2009, is currently developing a guide to help care partners and people with dementia address ethical dilemmas they might encounter. While general guidance is being established, the intricate and personal nature of dementia means that there are no definitive answers to the many complex and profound questions surrounding the ethical development and use of technology for supporting people living with dementia; rather, we need to leverage overarching principles to guide individuals' choices regarding appropriate technology use.

In this chapter, we will explore the role ethics plays in technology for people with dementia. The chapter starts with an overview of ethical principles before discussing how ethics can influence design and adoption of technology.

Ethical principles

In the context of this chapter, 'technology' is broadly defined to mean a device, system or intervention that enables people to achieve a desired goal. Technologies can play an important role in supporting social engagement, decision making and advance planning by individuals living with dementia (Alzheimer's Society 2017). Although technology can have considerable benefits, such as independence for persons with dementia, it also has potential negative aspects and the risk that it can be misused. For example, some technologies may intrude upon the rights, privacy and freedom of people living with dementia if they are not designed, adopted and used appropriately. Ethical principles and related concepts such as dignity, solidarity and autonomy are all relevant to the care and wellbeing of persons with dementia and their carers but also to other members of society such as the general public, device developers, service providers and policymakers (Godwin 2012; Hesook 2017).

Key moral ethical principles

One of the most widely used ethical frameworks is Beauchamp and Childress' (2009) four moral principles: non-maleficence, beneficence, autonomy and justice. While originally intended to guide biomedical ethics, they offer a broad consideration that has general applicability.

- *Non-maleficence* simply means 'do no harm', for example, considering whether there is a risk that using a technology may lead to additional confusion or distress for the person with dementia.

- *Beneficence* means striving consciously to be 'of benefit' to the person. The intention of an intervention or course of action should be to benefit the persons with dementia, for example by enabling access to support or help if they fall or helping them to take their medication. In addition, the World Health Organization (WHO 2017) requires that governments, healthcare providers and researchers do good for, provide benefit to, or make a positive contribution to the welfare of populations, patients and research participants.

- *Autonomy* refers to the ability of a person to be their own person and to make their own choices on the basis of their own motivations, without manipulation by external forces (WHO 2017). This corresponds to respecting a person's rights to self-determination, privacy, freedom and choice. Technologies can have a considerable effect on the lives of persons with dementia in terms of their autonomy and independence (Smebye, Kirkevold and Engedal 2016). For example, if a device such as a sensor mat is used to help monitor the risk of falls, would it just be used to tell the person not to walk or get up, or would the person be offered a companion to walk with safely? Also, certain types of tracking device cannot be easily removed, which means that once they have been put on, the person with dementia no longer has the freedom to take them off even if they want to, which violates their autonomy and ability to make their own choices.

- *Justice* means treating everyone fairly by equitably distributing risks, benefits and costs. All people have the right to be treated fairly, including people with dementia. This includes providing equal access to technology and accounting for diversity.

Informed consent

Informed consent in the context of dementia and technology means making sure that everyone using the technology understands the purpose, risks, benefits and alternative options for a technology in a way that enables them to make an informed choice about whether or not to use the technology. Consent is more than agreement to the use of assistive technology; consent means the person understands its function and freely agrees to engage with it. For example, a person with dementia who consents to wearing a bracelet without realising that it enables other people to monitor his or her whereabouts has not provided informed consent.

It is often assumed that people with dementia cannot give consent. In fact, the default position should be that people with dementia *can* give consent and that this should always be sought. Capacity to give consent is not something a person either has or does not have, rather it depends on the situation and how the issue is presented. Moreover, consent is not something that is given once, but should be considered an ongoing process; people have the right to change their mind.

Ideally, people who are responsible for obtaining consent for the use of devices or systems should be trained in appropriate communication methods for acquiring consent (Alzheimer Europe 2014). In some cases, people asking for consent may need to adapt the way they communicate so that people with dementia are able to give legally recognised consent. To do otherwise means that the rights of people with dementia are not being respected (Martin, Bengtsson and Dröes 2010). The question then is: How can people asking for consent adapt their approach to make it appropriate for people living with dementia?

The issue of informed consent when using technologies with people with dementia is complex (Novitzky *et al.* 2015). The capacity of a person with dementia to consent is likely to deteriorate over time and in some cases may fluctuate from day to day or at different times of the day. Alzheimer Europe (2010) and AT Dementia (2017) suggest using verbal and non-verbal approaches such as pictures, videos or demonstrations of the technology involved. This approach enables the person with dementia to leverage different communication methods as well as gain the confidence to engage in conversation or ask questions if he or she wishes to. In the cases of more advanced stages of dementia, making an effort to obtain consent as well as carefully monitoring the person for indications of assent or dissent are important to ensure technology is not causing frustration or distress.

Even after every effort has been made to obtain informed consent, a person may consent to the installation of surveillance equipment but later not be aware that they are being monitored or be able to reaffirm or withhold consent. When acquiring technology, consider thinking about how the technology would be uninstalled if the wishes or needs of a person with dementia change. Who would uninstall the product? Who would incur the costs? Essén (2008) emphasised the importance of having built-in possibilities to exit such services.

No one should be coerced into using technology, particularly technology that tracks or monitors a person's whereabouts. People with dementia should be involved in making decisions about technologies to use or not use. Where possible, people with dementia, their care partners and care professionals should make decisions together about the use of technology at the time of diagnosis (Meiland *et al.* 2017). These decisions can be made with the help of a professional team (Landau and Werner 2012). If someone with a cognitive impairment has been deemed not to have capacity to consent, a balance may be required between their right to autonomy and choice and the need to protect their safety and wellbeing. In this case, care partners and care professionals would be responsible for decision making.

There are various consent mechanisms that can be used by the person living with dementia giving consent when they have the mental capacity to do so. The concept of advance directives or 'living wills', sometimes called a Ulysses contract, is a binding directive provided by the person when they have the mental capacity to provide such a directive (Puran 2005). The directive is normally on aspects of future care, and in effect transfers decision making to a surrogate, for example, a caregiver.

Regardless, as the cognitive abilities of people with dementia can decline over time, it is important to reassess their capacity at regular intervals and to continue 're-informing' using appropriate reminders and updates. People living with dementia should have control over their consent in a way that enables them to autonomously change their mind whenever they wish, affording them the same rights as people who are deemed 'cognitively intact'. Related to this preservation of autonomy, it is important that the user or a proxy has full control of the technology so that the user's wishes can be acted upon in a timely manner.

Confidentiality and privacy

Confidentiality is the obligation to keep information private unless its disclosure has been appropriately authorised by the person concerned or, in extraordinary circumstances, by the appropriate authorities, such as the police (WHO 2017). The information gathered by technologies must be stored safely and used only for the purposes for which it was intended. There are important data protection issues around the use of assistive technologies, especially the use of telecare systems, and care must be taken to ensure that information gathered about a user is stored securely. If this information is being shared with other care professionals to help support the care planning process, procedures should be in place to ensure that this is done on a need-to-know basis only and solely for the purpose intended. At the moment, this is done on a case-by-case basis that is dependent upon the technology being used, who is providing the technology and who is using it.

As information technology (IT) use becomes the norm, privacy breaches and security threats are significant concerns. Informational privacy refers to the 'right of individuals to determine if, when, how and to what extent data about themselves will be collected, stored, transmitted, used and shared with others' (Cannon 2005, p.9). Security, on the other hand, is the set of mechanisms required to protect privacy (Cannon 2005). These concerns may be justified as technology development leads to advanced means for collecting and merging information about individuals, and therefore 'private spaces where individuals may remain free from intrusion seem to diminish' (Palm and Hansson 2006, p.553). For example, for persons with cognitive limitations, IT has been increasingly used to monitor their whereabouts through the use of tracking devices. While this form of IT use appears benevolent and useful (i.e. to protect the individual from getting lost or to help them learn to navigate their community; Stock *et al.* 2011), it may also represent a potential source of privacy intrusion and may lead to stigma associated with 'tagging' (Landau and Werner 2012; Niemeijer *et al.* 2013; Perry, Beyer and Holm 2009; Zwijsen, Niemeijer and Hertogh 2011). Indeed, persons with cognitive limitations might be discriminated against because such technology use emphasises their limitations, especially when using devices that are not used by persons without disabilities.

A study with people living with dementia, their families and healthcare professionals found that while those people living with dementia disliked remote monitoring and surveillance, their caregivers were pragmatic, prioritising safety (Godwin 2012). Kenner (2008, p.266) summarised this issue:

> exercising control over elderly people with dementia seems to be necessary and may be the best way to ensure wellbeing...if monitoring systems advance further understandings of dementia, help caregivers manage their responsibilities, and keep the elderly safe, how concerned should the public be about issues that have always plagued caregiving relations-control, privacy, autonomy, and power asymmetries?

Another example of possible intrusion is cloud computing services that reduce costs by sharing computing and storage resources (Pearson and Benameur 2010). This form of IT use may pose the risk of data being used by or stolen from service providers (Pearson and Benameur 2010).

Ethical design and use of technology

Can a technology or non-living thing be considered ethical or unethical? Is it the technology, the technology creator or its use that is considered ethical? Furthermore, who is responsible when the technology does not function as expected? Philosophical questions such as these underpin how we go about determining what constitutes ethical design and use of technology. One may argue that given the fact that technologies are currently insentient and not self-aware, technology itself is neither ethical nor unethical since it only functions according to its design (Singer 2011). This inherently transfers ethical considerations regarding technology to the people who decide how the technology is intended to function as well as how it is used. These ethical considerations become even more important when the technology is for a vulnerable user or a person living with dementia as they may not have the capacity to make fully informed choices regarding when and how it is used.

The use of technology to support people living with dementia has grown exponentially in the period 2012–2017, with an average five-year increase of 400 per cent in the use of 'intelligent assistive technology', i.e. 'technologies that sense and respond to user needs, are adaptable to changing situations and compensate either for physical or cognitive deficits' (Bharucha *et al.* 2009, p.102) in dementia care (Ienca *et al.* 2017). However, a literature review in the use of such technologies for the care of people with dementia has revealed that many of these technologies are designed in the absence of explicitly ethical values or considerations (Ienca *et al.* 2018). The norm to date has been the reactive use of ethical principles as a means of assessing the normative ethical 'positioning' of a technology in use by people living with dementia, normally against commonly used ethical principles such as autonomy, beneficence, non-maleficence and justice, which were discussed earlier in the chapter. Solutions resulting from reactive development are generally a poor fit to users' needs. Ienca and colleagues argue for a proactive approach that embeds ethical considerations in the design and development of new assistive technology products (Ienca *et al.* 2017), based upon a value-sensitive design approach which involves human values in a 'principled and comprehensive manner throughout the design process' (Friedman *et al.* 2013, p.1).

Often the developers of technologies used by people with dementia and their carers have designed with consideration only to the user needs of a broad population, and not specifically to address the identified needs of people living with dementia. Furthermore, even for technology-based products and services that have been specifically created for people with dementia, it is almost always the case that these designers receive no specialised training in ethical design principles or in understanding the needs of people with dementia. This means it is important to take time to check the credentials of product and service designers; perhaps check for evidence to see if they have gained endorsement from organisations such as the Alzheimer's Society or that their product or service has won a dementia-friendly design award.

It is not realistic to think that technology developers can anticipate, identify and deal with all the effects of their products, including privacy threats (Palm and Hansson 2006); however, adequate training could equip them to identify, from the start and throughout the technology development and commercialisation process, the benefits and potential negative consequences of IT use for different stakeholders (Balebako *et al.* 2014; Palm and Hansson 2006). Many authors agree that such training is simply missing (Balebako *et al.* 2014; Palm and Hansson 2006). If discussions around privacy and security threats were part of the design process from the start, 'there would be a greater chance for constructive interaction between social values and technological potential in which ethical problems could be dealt with at an early stage' (Palm and Hansson 2006, p.548; see also Cavoukian 2012).

Society, groups and individuals have a shared responsibility to manage the ethical uptake and use of technology.

Design thinking and user-centred design

Designing technology for people with dementia should be user-centred, meaning the prime consideration is how the technology interfaces with the person with dementia and their life. User-centred design approaches assume that the different needs of the people using technology-based products and services are front and centre in design thinking. As such, they adopt product and service design practices, including user-centred design, a well-established approach that puts the user at the centre of the design process (Rubin 1994), as well as other methods, such as cooperative design (Bødker 1993) and user experience (Norman, Miller and Henderson 1995). The key aim in these paradigms is to focus on the user's needs and experiences to create a product or service that is best suited to meet the needs of the user, with the intention of attaining better usability. Many of these concepts have also made their way into usability standards certified by the International Organization for Standardization,[1] the International Electrotechnical Commission[2] and the US Food and Drug Administration,[3] all of which are generally good indicators of best practice.

Privacy by design

The embedding of ethics into the design process borrows on the concept of privacy by design, a concept that entails embedding privacy into the design specifications of technologies. Privacy by design itself builds upon the principles of Fair Information Practices for the design, operation and management of information processing technologies and systems (Cavoukian 2011). The applicability of this approach when engineering systems does raise issues: deploying such methods might limit the utility of the resulting system (van Rest *et al.* 2012). This also builds on the concept of 'privacy by design' where the highest level of privacy is the default and users must opt out to lower levels of protection (Cavoukian 2011).

---

1   www.iso.org
2   www.iec.ch
3   www.fda.gov

Recent research has reported the absence, and therefore the need, for ethical considerations in the design and development of new technologies (Ienca *et al.* 2018; Meiland *et al.* 2017). Meiland and colleagues (2017) recommended developers take care to avoid replication of technology development that is unhelpful or ineffective; the focus should rather be on how technologies can support the individual needs of persons with dementia (Landau and Werner 2012; Meiland *et al.* 2017).

Ethical adoption of technology

Striking a proper balance between the ethical principles that are competing in this context is a shared responsibility of all stakeholders, including persons with cognitive limitations (Chalghoumi *et al.* 2017). Justice and beneficence should not overshadow the respect of the autonomy of persons with cognitive limitations; technologies should be accessible to them and lead to better outcomes, but first and foremost, should be integrated as part of the individual's supports after a decision-making process led by the person with cognitive limitations. Seale (2014) and Seale and Chadwick (2017) propose a 'positive risk-taking framework' that complements this ethical reflection. Based on two key components, shared decision making and risk management, this approach involves developing strategies so that the risks of an action are balanced against its benefits (Seale 2014; Seale and Chadwick 2017). This positive decision-making framework offers operational strategies and steps that may help take our reflection to a practical level: a shared decision-making process.

When considering using technologies for persons with dementia, an individualised, person-centred assessment of the need of the person with dementia and their informal carers should be carried out. Who does this and how it is done is dependent on the type of technology, the ability of the people using it and its intended use. Moreover, sometimes the needs of a person with dementia and their carer may differ or even conflict. Carers or others may overestimate the difficulties or risk to the person they care for. This can be a problem for practitioners trying to determine the extent of the person's difficulties or the level of risk to which they are exposed in the home and whether assistive technology has a role in managing these (Alzheimer Europe 2010;

Alzheimer's Society 2017). For example, one may need to decide whether to use a technology that might increase activity completion but takes away from what the person with dementia is still able to do for him or herself.

Considerations for adopting a technology

Several organisations – including Alzheimer Europe, the Alzheimer's Society and AT Dementia – have created guidelines and questions to help people make decisions about using technology with people with dementia. The *ASTRID Guide to Using Technology within Dementia Care* (Marshall 2000) is a resource developed by experts from the UK, Norway, the Netherlands and Ireland as part of the ASTRID project in response to meeting the needs of persons with dementia and their carers. Another helpful resource is 'The ethical use of assistive technology', a resource available on the AT Dementia website (AT Dementia 2017), which provides guidance based on Beauchamp and Childress' four ethical principles.

In addition to such resources, it can be helpful to use questions as a way to identify and think about information that is helpful to understanding and making decisions about whether and when to engage with technologies. Examples of such questions can be found in Box 3.1.

Box 3.1 Questions that can be used support the exploration and use of technologies

Questions that could be asked when considering whether to use technology:

- What is the problem that you're trying to solve?

- What action has been tried to solve the problem?

- Does the situation require technology? Are there alternatives to using technology?

- What technology options are available that might help solve the problem?

Questions to ask when evaluating a technology:

- What would I want for myself in this situation?

- Are there risks associated with using the technology? What are the risks? Are they real risks or perceived risks?

- What are the benefits of the technology for both the person with dementia and the care partners? What are the drawbacks?

- Would the technology help the person do things that they might not be able to do otherwise (for example, connect with loved ones, carry out a task or remember events)?

- What are the consequences of using or not using the technology?

Questions to ask when adopting a technology:

- Has the person with dementia given informed consent? Does the person understand the purpose, risks and benefits of the technology?

- Have you considered what will happen if the person with dementia changes their mind about the technology? Who will uninstall it? Who will pay for any costs associated with uninstalling it?

Holistic care approach

Alzheimer Europe's (2014) report highlighted a more holistic care approach to ethics, which takes into consideration the whole person (i.e. their uniqueness, their relationships to others and their dignity and vulnerability) as well as their unique situation. This ethical approach is based on the work of Gastmans (2013) and incorporates the role of conscience developed by Hughes and Baldwin (2006). The main features of Alzheimer Europe's approach include: the lived experience; the interpretive dialogue; a normative standard reflecting vulnerability, dignity, interdependency and relationships; and our informed conscience. The report provides a step-by-step approach to everyday ethical dilemmas that is intended to provide a structure to help address relevant issues for all who are involved (Box 3.2).

Box 3.2 Step-by-step approach to address relevant issues in everyday ethical dilemmas

1. Establish and maintain an ongoing dialogue with everyone involved or concerned about the particular issue.

2. Try to understand the issue and seek additional information if needed.

3. Try to make sense of people's needs, wishes and concerns (i.e. what is really important to them or bothering them).

4. Consider and evaluate the ethical principles and values at stake in relation to the individuals involved (including yourself) and the specific situation.

5. Reflect together on possible outcomes which might be good or bad for different people concerned, bearing in mind their lived experiences.

6. Take a stance, act accordingly and, bearing in mind that you did your best, try to come to terms with the outcome.

7. Reflect on the resolution of the dilemma and what you have learnt from the experience.

Case studies

The following case studies are about real-world examples of different technologies to illustrate how some of the themes discussed above have been considered and put into practice.

Case study 3.1 MemorySparx by Emmetros

MemorySparx is a digital memory aid designed to support people with early- to mid-stage dementia. It works on an iPad and helps people with memory loss organise and recall information about their day, their life and their health through photos, notes and voice recordings. MemorySparx is designed by Emmetros, a technology company committed to helping people with cognitive impairment live with independence and dignity; screenshots with examples of tasks supported by MemorySparx can be seen in Figure 3.1. Initially, the Emmetros team intended to create a digital memory aid that a family member or care partner would populate on behalf of a person with dementia. When they talked with people with dementia, though, the team discovered that many wanted to have the ability to add and manage content themselves. Consequently, the team shifted their focus. They worked with people with dementia to design a tool that would work for them and give them the autonomy they sought.

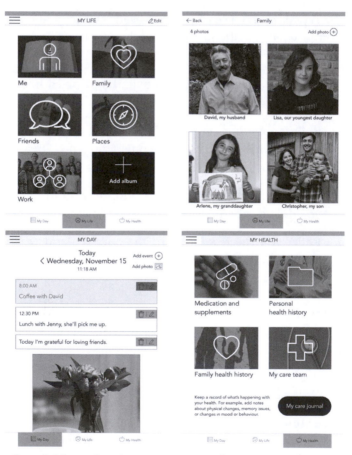

Figure 3.1 Screenshots demonstrating some of MemorySparx's functions (clockwise from top left): 'My Life' homepage, 'Family', 'My Health' and 'My Day'

The Emmetros team believe that engaging people living with dementia and keeping their needs at the centre of the design process results in better, more usable and useful products. Engaging people with dementia helps the team understand what people love about MemorySparx (what excites and delights them) as well as how the product can be improved to better equip people to mitigate the challenges they face every day.

To support their user-centred approach, Emmetros developed an engagement model that involves the following key user experience (UX) activities:

Interviews or 'meet and greets'

When Emmetros connects with a person with dementia, a UX researcher from the team conducts a 'meet and greet' interview with that person and their care partner (if the person with dementia would like a care partner present). This interview allows everyone to get to know each other and gives the UX researcher a chance to share information about design and development activities the person might be interested in participating in. To help people with dementia and their care partners feel safe and comfortable, these interviews are conducted in a location and at a time that the person with dementia chooses.

Exploratory research and usability studies

During exploratory research sessions or usability sessions, a UX researcher from the Emmetros team asks people with dementia to explore MemorySparx and complete tasks. He or she talks with them about their experience and observes them for signs of confusion or frustration. The UX researcher emphasises throughout these sessions that the person with dementia is the expert and that there's no such thing as a silly question or a wrong answer.

Design walkthroughs

Emmetros also conducts design walkthroughs with care partners. During a design walkthrough, a UX researcher from the team shows care partners design concepts and asks them for candid and honest feedback. This feedback informs enhancements to the product to make it more beneficial for people with dementia and, by extension, their care partners.

Product testing

For product testing, Emmetros provides MemorySparx to people with dementia for a period of four to six weeks. Participants have a chance to use the app at their own pace. No pressure. A UX researcher from the Emmetros team follows up with them regularly (typically once a week) to discover what they're doing with the product and how they feel about the experience. All product testers are free to use the app whenever and however they see fit, at times that are convenient for them.

Follow-up meetings

As much as possible, the Emmetros team follow up with people who participate in usability studies and product testing to let them know how their contributions informed changes to the product. The team want people with dementia and their care partners to know that their efforts have impact.

For all UX activities, Emmetros attains informed, written consent from all participants. All consent forms for participants are written in plain language in short, clear sections to support understanding. The Emmetros team sends the forms in advance of any interaction, giving people with dementia and their care partners time to process the information and formulate questions. Then at the beginning of an interaction (typically a face-to-face interaction), a UX researcher verbally reviews the forms to make sure that everyone understands and is comfortable with the terms. At that time, the UX researcher also let participants know that they're free to withdraw from any activity at any time – no questions asked.

All research data and personal information Emmetros collects from people with dementia and their care partners is kept confidential and is used only by the product development team to inform product design. In their privacy policy, Emmetros clearly explains, in plain language, that protection of people's personal information is a top priority. MemorySparx users and testers own the information they add to the app, and Emmetros does everything they can to keep that information secure (for example, storing personal information in an encrypted form on professionally managed services located in secure storage facilities). The Emmetros team understands they are working with personal information from a vulnerable group, and they are committed to preserving people's privacy and safety.

As the Emmetros team tries things out and learns about what works well and what doesn't work as well when engaging people with dementia, they want others to learn too – so much so that they recently partnered with the University of Waterloo and the Murray Alzheimer Research and Education Program (MAREP) on an 18-month research project exploring best practices for engaging people with dementia respectfully and meaningfully in design and testing of technology intended for their use, as reflected in Figure 3.2. By sharing what they learn, the Emmetros team hope to influence other product developers who are creating technology for people with dementia to take a user-centred, ethical approach to their work.

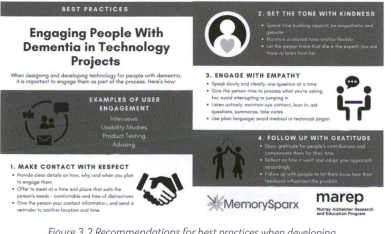

Figure 3.2 Recommendations for best practices when developing technology for and with people living with dementia

(Reproduced with permission of Emmetros Limited and the Murray Alzheimer Research and Education Programme (MAREP))

Case study 3.2 Video surveillance at home

This case study reports on the issues around the use of video surveillance in the home from the perspectives of people living with dementia and their carers. The case study presents the feedback from workshops in 2014 where Age Northern Ireland (AgeNI) facilitated the event in Northern Ireland at which Ulster University academics gathered the views of the participants.

The rationale for the workshops was to elicit the views of both those who could be the focus of surveillance and their carers, to examine if the literature supported their views and to discuss the findings from the literature with this study group. In total, 24 participants took part in this study, consisting of two persons living with dementia and 22 caregivers. As part of the workshop, the participants were asked to respond using a questionnaire which explored issues surrounding the use of video cameras in caring for a person living with dementia. The results indicated that 91 per cent thought that the idea of a video camera in the home of a person living with dementia living alone was a very good or good idea, while 92 per cent thought that the concept was very appropriate or appropriate, dropping to 78 per cent considering it very appropriate or appropriate for use in homes of older people generally.

Beauchamp and Childress' (2009) four ethical principles of autonomy, beneficence, non-maleficence and justice were reflected in the written responses of participants in the workshops in many cases, with many presenting arguments and reflections around the net benefit of beneficence with non-maleficence. The principle that presented most frequently related to autonomy, both from the perspectives of people living with dementia:

'If properly placed being mindful of privacy it allows the person to live at home for longer and remain independent'

and from the carers' perspective:

'It relieves the anxiety of the family who are concerned about the safety of the person with dementia and it affords those who are caring for a person with dementia more freedom.'

The general sentiment from participants can be illustrated in the following quotes:

'Because it would give me assurance that Mum goes to bed. Also to monitor her movements as she won't wear a telecare bracelet.'

'If managed appropriately, I feel that this concept could enable someone with dementia to remain at home for longer. Respecting the individual rights is paramount and this concerns me. I think education and demonstration would be beneficial.'

'If used properly, this could provide great support for those with dementia, provide comfort for those who are caring for them and provide valuable insight into the behaviours that those with dementia exhibit. It could allow relatives living abroad the opportunity of being involved in caring for someone with dementia; like speed cameras, they can change the behaviours of people. Carers who know and are aware of the presence of a camera will afford the person the correct amount of time being paid for and deliver a better quality of care.'

'Mainly safety, and peace of mind for family.'

There were also more cautious perspectives from participants, for example:

'Monitoring safety, mobility, bringing peace of mind to carers. Must be suitable circumstances, respecting necessary privacy with proper permissions and for right reasons.'

'For me it is about the ethics and safeguarding of the vulnerable person. I believe that there are some merits, but I am not totally convinced but can understand that families directly involved would have perhaps divergent views.'

'If it is limited to movement and hallways I would be more comfortable but in living rooms, bedrooms, you are taking away human rights – big issue. Everyone is an individual – even with dementia.'

'Proper consent from person needs to be sought so that they feel comfortable with this method. System needs to be independent from other government bodies. Only family have access. Should be used by family to eliminate any worries and to identify any support needs to benefit from the care package for the person.'

The families who participated in the workshops outlined different perceived effects of video surveillance, including financial protection, privacy, security, safety and peace of mind. They were generally supportive of the concept of the use of camera in the homes of people living with dementia, with some significant caveats. The use of cameras in the home of a person living with dementia where family caregivers could monitor their family member with dementia was supported as useful, ethical and moral providing the right protocol is in place to gain consent. However, when professional caregivers are involved (e.g. as part of the care team) and therefore one of the people 'observed' by the camera or as part of the authorised 'observation team', then the degree of ethical discomfort increases.

Gaps and areas for future development

The ethical use of technology is and will continue to be a complex and crucial matter that requires active input ranging from society in general to the person with dementia it is intended to support. Decisions regarding the use of technologies and implementing their uses, who partakes in these decisions and who is ultimately responsible should consider the ethical issues from the perspectives of the person with dementia, family caregivers and professional providers, and it should only be used when it is needed and wanted. For example, emerging health-related technologies can pose new and significant risks. In assessing those risks, the focus is often on social acceptance, however, social acceptance studies do not adequately capture the morally relevant characteristics of these technologies. Studies of ethical acceptability may not include stakeholder perspectives and consequently they may not permit a complete evaluation of ethical issues.

It is only when perspectives from as many viewpoints as possible are examined, considered, discussed and addressed that we can trend towards ethical decision making. As such, each person's individual needs, context and values must be taken into account when weighing up the pros and cons of any device. In the case of technology for supporting someone living with dementia, this includes being clear about the purpose of the technology and how the person with dementia, their family and their care partners may or may not benefit from it and how they can truly make the choice whether or not to engage with the technology. Just as important is supporting people's ability to *disengage* with a technology: to have the freedom and ability to choose not to continue using a technology should they wish to do so.

While work has been done in this area, as the capabilities and uses of technologies continue to expand and change, practitioners, policymakers, care insurers, care providers and people with dementia themselves must work together with technology enterprises and researchers to guide the ethical development, implementation and use of technologies.

Take-home points

The ethical design, uptake and use of technology for supporting dementia must include the following:

* *Respect autonomy and independence:* The needs of the person with dementia are paramount in deciding if and what devices should be used for them. Carers and practitioners need to be clear that there are legitimate reasons to employ technologies and should provide everyone involved with the most freedom possible; this includes the freedom to choose whether or not to engage or disengage with a technology.

* *Decision-making and informed consent must be accessible to everyone:* Persons with dementia and their families should be fully informed about and consent to the use of technologies. When choosing to use technology, the person with dementia must be centrally involved in deciding to do so, and their consent must be sought and gained to the greatest extent possible. In cases where decisions need to be made in the person's best interests, they should be considerate of the individual's rights and must be the least restrictive option. Care and consideration are needed in relation to how information is provided to enable them to make an informed choice. If the person does have capacity and does not consent to the use of assistive technology, their decision must be respected.

* *Uphold wellbeing:* The safety and wellbeing of the person with dementia should be paramount. Technology cannot replace human contact and should never be used as a substitute for proper social care. People making the decisions regarding the use of technology need to consider and weigh the benefits and the risks to themselves as well as the person with dementia.

* *Periodically revisit decisions:* Situations and needs change; what may have been the right choice at one point may no longer be the best option. Decisions regarding the use or non-use of technology should be periodically revisited to ensure all concerned parties are in agreement.

PART 2

Technology in the Lives of People with Dementia

Chapter 4

Life at Home and Technology with Dementia

Dr Grant Gibson, *Lecturer in Dementia Studies, University of Stirling, UK*

Introduction

Enabling people with dementia to live independently in their own homes is a key objective of contemporary dementia care policy and practice. Frequently referred to as 'ageing in place', current healthcare policy across many western countries focuses upon ensuring people with dementia can stay at home as their dementia progresses, thereby delaying, reducing or avoiding the use of state services such as residential or nursing care (Brittain *et al.* 2010; Buffel, Phillipson and Scharf 2012; Kenner 2008; Roberts, Mort and Milligan 2012). Such policy objectives typically have the support of older people themselves, with the majority routinely stating that they would prefer to remain at home for as long as possible (Lui *et al.* 2009; Oldman 2003). In order to support this objective, assistive technologies have been posited as a means to support people with dementia to remain at home (Sixsmith and Sixsmith 2008). Products defined as assistive technology can include a whole range of mobility aids and household adaptations; however, in the context of people living with dementia, the term 'assistive technology' is most often associated with electronic devices or services which can monitor a person's activities, or products that can assist a person with daily functions (Gibson *et al.* 2016).

This chapter explores how technologies can be used to support people with dementia in the home, alongside some of the issues that emerge when technologies are used to help care for people at home. The chapter discusses some of the main uses of assistive technology around the home, as well as reviewing the range and remit of technologies that are currently available. Case study examples of technologies and services emerging from research with people with dementia also show how technologies can support people with dementia living at home. Additionally, these cases explore how people with dementia and their carers interact with and use these technologies in the home. Finally, the chapter concludes with a discussion of how a number of new technologies, including smartphone and tablet-based apps, and smart home technologies, will support people with dementia to live at home in the near future.

Assistive technology and the home

Assistive technology in dementia covers a wide gamut of devices and products. These range from complex networks of devices such as telecare, through the 'Internet of Things', or smart home and mobile technologies embedded within everyday devices which are able to send and receive data from each other via the Internet, down to simple objects such as cutlery and crockery, or using paper notes to provide instructions, prompts or reminders (Gibson *et al.* 2016). Indeed, simple adaptations such as putting instructions on devices or covering buttons with tape are some of the most common ways in which technology is used to help with care (Gibson *et al.* 2015; Greenhalgh *et al.* 2013). Given both the rapid pace of technological development and the increasing political focus on providing care from a distance there is unsurprisingly an expanding range of technologies aimed at older people and people with dementia. However, this 'mixed economy' comprising public and commercial providers can be confusing, with awareness of devices, people's ability to access them, the range of devices on offer and their associated cost often varying according to where you live, the services available to you or your ability to pay (Newton *et al.* 2016).

Most assistive technologies used in dementia have focused on improving safety and security, thereby reducing the risks people with dementia may face at home. Such technologies typically take the form of 'telecare': suites of sensors connected via a phone link or Internet connection to either informal carers or social care services. It is important to note, however, that the use of technology in dementia care is not limited to safety, security and the mitigation of risk. People with dementia frequently have difficulties with everyday tasks around the home. For example, they may struggle to use everyday objects such as kitchen equipment, telephones, televisions or remote controls. This leads to difficulties with cooking and household activities, taking part in leisure activities or keeping in touch with family or friends (Nygård 2008). Such problems are powerful determinants of whether a person with dementia can remain at home, meaning that any assistance with them can enable people to stay independent for longer (Nygård and Starkhammar 2007).

Technology can also improve social participation for people with dementia, by ensuring home environments are 'dementia friendly', by enabling people to maintain social contact with friends or family or by giving people access to enjoyable activities such as music, physical activity or games (Sixsmith and Gibson 2007; Wherton and Monk 2008; Zheng, Chen and Yu 2017). For example, music players with a minimum number of controls can give people with dementia at home easy access to music (see Example 4.1).

Example 4.1 Simple Music Player

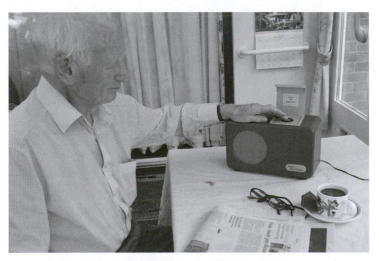

Figure 4.1 Person using the Simple Music Player

The Simple Music Player emerged from research funded by the UK Engineering and Physical Sciences Research Council (EPSRC) which sought to develop assistive technologies that could promote quality of life by enabling access to enjoyable activities (Orpwood *et al.* 2010; Sixsmith and Gibson 2007). A series of qualitative research interviews with people with dementia and their carers highlighted both the importance of music, and also the difficulties people had in using common music players. The proposed solution involved a simple, one-button music player, in a form factor which looked broadly similar to a radio, but which also clearly communicated its control mechanisms. Several years after the research concluded a technology company licenced the specification. Following several further design iterations, the company developed a commercial version, which is now available online and in UK high street stores.

In a review of assistive technology products available in the UK, Gibson *et al.* (2016) identified 171 different technologies and technology types across 11 domains (see Figure 4.2). Given the rapid pace of development, this number will already be out of date as more products enter the market. The typology proposed by Gibson *et al.* (2016) classifies technologies according to who uses them and how they are used. Technologies used 'by' a person with dementia are typically designed for the person to interact with directly and are associated with household tasks within the home such as cooking or using the bathroom, or provide easier access to entertainment, communication and leisure. Examples include television remote controls, clocks, prompting devices, simple signs, kitchen timers and reminder alarms. Devices used 'with' a person with dementia typically promote social interaction and participation. Examples of communication aids include telephones, mobile phones, video phones or video conferencing products. Several products promote social activities using simple or complex puzzles and games, or are aids to reminiscence using historic mock-ups of household products or using video, music and games. Exemplified by telecare, the third and most common classification of technologies are those used 'on' a person with dementia. Such technologies are typically passive systems installed in the home, which require little to no direct input from a person, but can raise an alarm in an emergency. Other devices include Global Positioning System (GPS) monitors, which can locate a person who has become lost; fall detectors, which raise an alarm after a fall; or telephone call blockers, which restrict nuisance telephone calls. These devices arguably hold the needs of formal and informal caregivers as their primary concern, rather than the needs of the person with dementia (Mort, Roberts and Callen 2013).

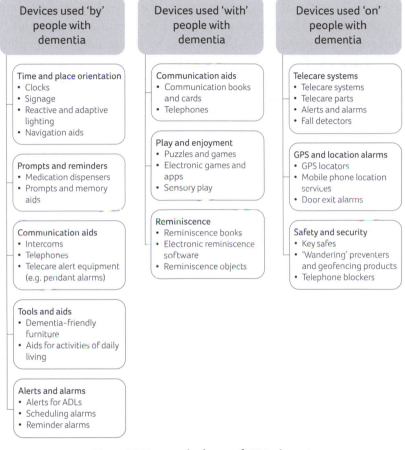

Figure 4.2 Types and subtypes of AT in dementia
(Gibson et al. 2016, used with permission)

In the UK, most assistive technology products are accessed through local authority social care services, and less often through health services such as occupational therapy. Although most devices are provided through health and social care services, a growing number of assistive products are also commercially available outside health and social care, leading to the development of a mixed economy for assistive technologies (Gibson *et al.* 2016). In practice, this market also contains a range of everyday, commercially available products which can also be used to fulfil a range of assistive function. Such functions may include simple adaptations such as hiding controls with tape through to video conferencing via software tools such as Skype or FaceTime to keep in touch with geographically dispersed family and friends (Gibson *et al.* 2015; Greenhalgh *et al.* 2013; Rosenberg and Nygård 2012). The commercial smart home sector, which includes sensors and cameras, can also be used to create bespoke versions of telecare which completely bypass health and social care services (Gibson *et al.* 2015). As a generation of older people who are more comfortable with such technologies begin to experience dementia, this mixed economy of technology-enabled care, in which people can (and in many cases have to) buy commercial products and services alongside those provided by statutory services, will grow both in its social significance and its commercial potential.

Telecare and living with dementia at home

When considering the role of technology in dementia care, technology developers, health and social care providers and policymakers have undoubtedly paid greatest attention to telecare. With its origins in the community alarm systems that have become ubiquitous in supported housing, the past ten years have seen telecare become a mainstream part of dementia care provision across several developed nations. European countries adopting telecare at scale include the UK (Bowes and McColgan 2013; Gibson *et al.* 2015; Orpwood *et al.* 2010; Robinson *et al.* 2009), Spain (Lopez-Gomez 2015; Lopez-Gomez and Sanchez-Criado 2009), Sweden (Rosenberg and Nygård 2012), Norway (Arntzen, Holthe and Jentoft 2016), Germany (Megges *et al.* 2017) and the Netherlands (Pols and Moser 2009). In the UK context, programmes put into place to promote telecare more widely have included Building Telecare in England (Department of Health 2005), Delivering Assisted Living Devices at Scale (DALLAS),[1] launched in 2011, and '3 Million Lives',[2] while assistive technology plays a prominent role in both the UK Prime Minister's Challenge

---

1   www.dhaca.org.uk
2   www.3millionlives.co.uk; Woolham, Gibson and Clarke (2006).

for Dementia (Department of Health 2015) and the Third Scottish Dementia Strategy (Scottish Government 2017).

While configurations vary according to country, provider and service, a typical telecare system will comprise a suite of movement, temperature, flood and other sensors, connected to each other and to family carers and/or a monitoring centre via a wired or wireless network and broadband Internet connection. In the event of an emergency the system can identify such an event and alert a designated emergency contact such as a carer, family member, formal care service or the emergency services. More recent developments in telecare have focused on detailed lifestyle monitoring, which can detect even subtle changes in activities, behaviour or biometric data which over time may indicate that a problem is developing. For example, such technologies could potentially detect if a person is moving around the home more or less than usual, if medications are being missed or if blood pressure changes significantly, and can issue an alert if measures fall outside of a predetermined set of norms. An example lifestyle monitoring service is 'Canary'.[3] Canary measures a person's movements around the home, transmitting this information to family members or health professionals via an online interface. Significantly, Canary is available both through health and social care, and for private purchase, with direct sales forming a small but growing proportion of its sales.

The attention given to telecare is largely due to assumptions that by reducing the risks associated with ageing in place with dementia, telecare can enable people to remain at home for longer (Mort *et al.* 2013). In doing so the risks associated with living at home can be managed, delivering greater efficiencies and cost savings in the face of both a declining carer workforce and a growing population of older people with complex healthcare needs (Mort *et al.* 2013; Woolham *et al.* 2006). However, the current research evidence supporting these assumptions as gained from large-scale empirical studies is modest, with the data not necessarily supporting these assumptions (Greenhalgh *et al.* 2013, 2017). The Whole System Demonstrator (WSD) trial, a large-scale UK study of telecare and the largest in the world at the time, found that when used to treat a number of chronic conditions (including diabetes and heart failure but not dementia), telecare did not necessarily lead to improved outcomes, greater efficiencies or significant

---

3   www.canarycare.co.uk

cost savings, meaning telecare should not be seen as a 'magic bullet' (Henderson *et al.* 2014; Steventon *et al.* 2013).

The results of the Whole System Demonstrator led to much controversy and debate about the role of telecare in delivering care at home, and in the role of users in the process of mainstreaming telecare services. One side of the debate claimed that the evidence base for these technologies is unproven and that development of telecare services should be tempered by the need for evidence of their effectiveness. In contrast the other side claimed that flaws in the trial-based methodology, including low recruitment rates and take-up of devices, alongside a need for standardised services make it impossible to ascertain the effectiveness of complex interventions such as telecare using trial-based research (Greenhalgh 2012). Furthermore, as the utopian argument goes, as yet unknown evolutions in technology will enable both greater savings and more appropriate care as the technology is scaled up. Indeed, since the WSD trial ended in 2013 there has been an explosion of mainstream consumer devices based around smartphones, tablets, the Internet of Things and the existence of 'big data', each of which can conceivably turn dementia care on its head, although how far they can meet this potential is currently unknown. Where specific research on the role of telecare in dementia care has taken place, these have been limited to small-scale trials and pilot studies of individual devices. However, a number of large-scale UK-based projects, including 'Assistive technology and telecare to maintain independent living at home for people with dementia' (ATTILA), the Technology Integrated Health Management (TIHM) for dementia project and the Digital Support Platform (DSP) are in the process of reporting their findings (Dixon 2016; Killin *et al.* 2018; Leroi *et al.* 2013). Despite these debates regarding the efficacy of technologies, policy goals continue to 'mainstream' telecare as a part of care, meaning that these technologies will play at least some role in the future delivery of health and social care services for people with dementia at home.

Experiences of using technology in the home

Our homes are being filled with an ever-growing range of technologies, a trend likely to grow apace as the wave of interconnected 'smart home' technologies comes to fruition. Everyday services such as banking and shopping, as well as state services, such as pensions, benefits and health or social care services, are becoming more and more dependent on access to information and communication technologies. Yet despite the increasing penetration of technology into everyday life, in practice we know surprisingly little about how people with dementia make use of these technologies in their home environments, the challenges they face when doing so and how technology might best overcome those challenges (Gibson *et al.* 2015; Milligan, Roberts and Mort 2011; Nygård and Starkhammar 2007). The proliferation of many household technologies, alongside perceived, stereotypical and often ageist assumptions that older people are ambivalent regarding technologies, can mean that many technologies are not designed for older people, including people with dementia, to use (Gibson *et al.* 2015; Selwyn *et al.* 2003). How people use technologies will clearly be influenced by their dementia, but research has not yet adequately explored what factors contribute to the adoption, non-adoption or rejection of technologies, particularly as people move through the dementia journey (Greenhalgh *et al.* 2017).

Although the symptoms of dementia will clearly impact on a person's ability to use technology, this ability is also mediated by the design of products, including how well they fit into the home environment (Milligan *et al.* 2011; Orpwood *et al.* 2010). Nygård and Starkhammar (2007) describe people's ability to use technologies being reduced by their cognitive impairment. Crucially however, they also identify design issues limiting their usability as posing the greatest barriers to the successful use of technologies in the home (Gibson *et al.* 2016). Such design factors include the complexity of controls built into a device, how clearly a device communicates its purpose and how it should be used, and the inappropriate replacement of existing devices with new technology. Sensitive designs can overcome these problems, while insensitive designs, when combined with the inappropriate use of technologies, can create or accelerate dependency. For example, a person facing difficulties with cooking may find their family giving them a microwave oven to cook their meals, believing this will be easier to manage. However, a person's relative unfamiliarity with this technology may mean the microwave is not used, with the person instead relying on cold meals such as sandwiches. Such a solution, while well meaning, could well reduce nutritional intake, increase incapacity, and ultimately contribute to a move into assisted living earlier than necessary. This is not to suggest that all such interventions are wrong. However, difficulties with using technology cannot therefore simply be attributed to cognitive impairment; consideration of the inclusive design of technologies, the organisations providing them and the spaces in which technologies are located is necessary if technologies are to be implemented in ways that are sensitive to an individual's needs (Mort *et al.* 2015; Orpwood *et al.* 2007).

A regular feature of assistive technology provision is that it is introduced as a response to a crisis, after which a person poses too great a risk to remain at home without support (Toot *et al.* 2013). Examples of crises may include having a fall, getting lost when away from the home or causing a fire or flood through leaving items (e.g. a stove or tap) unattended. These events may necessitate an increase in the care offered to an individual or admission into residential or nursing care. However, the introduction of many assistive technologies as a response to a crisis may well be too late. It is preferable for technologies to be implemented as part of a proactive and preventive approach, in which potential future problems are recognised and assistance provided while people are able to learn and adapt to the technology. Unfortunately, the evidence suggests that for many services this is not routine practice (Milligan *et al.* 2011; Zwijsen *et al.* 2011). The issue is further complicated by research which suggests that many carers and people with dementia will resist the introduction of technologies if they do not think they are needed (Gibson *et al.* 2016; Killin *et al.* 2018). Therefore, if technology-enabled care services are to move away from a crisis- and deficits-based approach, new ways of thinking about both how services provide technologies and how technologies are designed and used are required.

That said, there are examples of services taking a more preventive and enabling approach to technology implementation. A now long-standing telecare project in West Lothian in Scotland developed a pioneering approach by offering telecare to every household containing residents over 60 years of age, instead of just those with health problems (including dementia; Bowes and McColgan 2006, 2013). This service also sought to give people the ability to make decisions autonomously, while being supported to do so by technology. Such an approach, in which telecare was truly mainstreamed, reduced the stigma which may be associated with requiring assistance and therefore being incapable, while also promoting a stronger sense of citizenship and social participation through the technology (Bowes and McColgan 2013).

Research exploring how people with dementia use telecare in the home has also indicated that technologies work best when they are introduced into a person's life in a way which is sensitive to the person's individual living situations and personal preferences (Bowes and McColgan 2013; Gibson *et al.* 2016). For example, a commonality across many studies of telecare systems is that many older people dislike wearing pendant alarms (Mort *et al.* 2013). Reasons for refusing to wear pendant alarms have been linked to memory difficulties, including forgetting to wear the device or forgetting what it does. However, people also frequently describe pendants getting in the way of their activities, or feeling that they don't need the pendant or that the pendants are stigmatising, for example labelling them as frail, vulnerable or incompetent (Lopez-Gomez 2015). For others, the alarms and alerts associated with pendant alarms and other telecare devices could be frightening if alarms were triggered accidentally or without the person's knowledge. In a recent study by Gibson *et al.* (2015), one woman living with dementia described her feelings about her pendant alarm:

> I'll tell you the truth, I'm terrified of it. When we first got it, it was over there and I didn't know what it was, and I happened to go over and I touched it and I thought, 'What is it?' Of course, the voice came up straight away, 'What's the matter?' It must go to a centre, some centre. And I said, 'Oh I'm sorry, I must've touched something.' (Gibson *et al.* 2015, p.7)

Clear ethical questions therefore emerge about the implementation of technology in and around the home, and what its consequences for a person's sense of home may be. Such questions include who technology is working for, and how far people have to reorder their homes and their lives, if technology is to work for them (Milligan *et al.* 2011). If technologies are to be successfully introduced, they must be sensitive to such issues.

Many people with dementia and their carers also use assistive technologies in the home in creative, personalised ways, which can vary significantly when compared to device designs (Mort *et al.* 2013).

For example, in a study by Gibson *et al.* (2016) people described finding alternative, often creative ways of using pendant alarms; rather than wearing them around their neck, people hung them over a lamp, placed them on a bedside cabinet or table by a chair, or carried them in a pocket. Such forms of use are not working from the perspective of the design of the pendant, or from the point of view of the service. But they are 'working' in at least some capacity for the person; they integrated technology into their lives in ways that were acceptable to them. Milligan *et al.* (2011), Roberts *et al.* (2012) and Lopez *et al.* (2009) also describe people 'misusing' pendant alarm by pressing the emergency button to speak to call centre workers for social contact. How services respond to this 'problem' varied; Roberts *et al.* (2012) describe some services removing systems, while Procter *et al.* (2016) in contrast described teleoperators chatting to users who had activated the alarm to find out if they were lonely. Describing similar findings, Lopez *et al.* (2009) and Mort *et al.* (2015) found that many teleoperators supported these social contacts against the instructions of management. Such research illustrates the emotional importance of technology-enabled care services providing what Pols and Moser (2009) call 'warm' care; new forms of care that, while technologically mediated, also foster social and emotional connections between services and their users. However, such 'warm' care may come into conflict with the organisational goals for telecare, such as increasing efficiency of care contacts, raising further questions about precisely who technology-enabled care services are working for: the person or the service itself (Mort *et al.* 2013).

The success or failure of many technologies in the home are also dependent on what Lopez-Gomez (2015) calls 'little arrangements': the various social and spatial arrangements necessary if technologies are to be used successfully. In a further research example, a woman with dementia living with her daughter used a GPS location monitor (Gibson *et al.* 2016). Sourced by her daughter, the GPS meant her mother's location could be monitored when she was outside, giving her a means to travel around on her own. Its use was supported by a series of habitual actions carried out by both the mother and daughter. The daughter retrieved the GPS from her mother's handbag each day, then placed it in a cradle to charge overnight. Each morning the GPS was placed in the same place: on a sideboard in the living room where the mother knew to find it. Through continued reinforcement, this sequence of actions had become part of the mother's daily routine. Indeed, the mother eventually forgot what the GPS was for, but still picked it up each morning. This GPS example demonstrates the complex but often hidden array of activities that are required to ensure that technologies in the home 'work'. Such arrangements are fundamental to the successful use of technology in the home, meaning services and devices must be sensitive to these arrangements when introducing technology into the home.

New technologies, dementia and the home

Recent years have seen a number of new technological developments and it is likely that such developments will continue, leading to important shifts in how care is provided to people with dementia at home (Sharkey and Sharkey 2014). Perhaps the technologies having greatest influence on 21st-century social life have been mobile computing using tablet computers and smartphones. Containing many times more processing power than the computers that sent people to the moon, smartphones are readily accessible at ever-reducing prices. While the latest versions cost several hundreds or even thousands of pounds, powerful smartphones can be bought at low cost. In addition, mobile and smartphones specifically targeted at older people and people with dementia are available, sold by companies such as Doro.[4] Importantly, smartphones contain the constituent parts of several assistive technologies, such as GPS monitors or accelerometers, and can easily be linked to external sensors or cameras, as well as using easily adaptable interfaces. Older people are a growing market for smartphones, with research indicating that approximately 71 per cent of UK adults over the age of 55 own one (Deloitte 2017). These figures suggest that the number of older people, including people with dementia, who are using smartphones and related technology is growing, with many older people having at least some knowledge of their capabilities.

Growing from now ubiquitous smartphones is the interface between smartphones, apps and a wide variety of smart home technologies. Known colloquially as the 'Internet of Things', two of the most common aspects of smart home technologies are their ability

---

4   www.doro.co.uk

to communicate with each other, and to be controlled remotely via smartphone applications or 'apps'. Using touchscreen technologies, well-designed apps can be inherently intuitive in their designs, so dementia need not necessarily pose a problem in terms of interacting with devices (Hernandez, Astell and Theiventhiran 2017; Joddrell, Hernandez and Astell 2016). With sensitive designs, smartphones and other everyday technologies therefore provide a number of assistive functions for people with dementia. Perhaps more importantly, they can also give people the opportunity to engage in meaningful social interaction, entertainment and leisure. The development of smartphones and apps means future iterations of assistive technology will look less like the fixed hardware installations of the past, instead becoming software solutions using existing, often portable and adaptable devices. Developments in voice recognition, such as Google's Home, Amazon's Alexa, Apple's Siri and Microsoft's Cortana, mean these could conceivably be used by a person with dementia to more easily control aspects of their home. Siri or Alexa will never become annoyed or angry, no matter how many times it is asked what time it is. Largely due to the newness of the technology, few studies currently exist at the time of writing which explore the applicability and usability of these platforms in dementia, or indeed what happens to the vast amounts of data they collect. However, anecdotal accounts of their use (e.g. Daily Caring 2017; Medium 2017) suggest that these technologies at least have the potential to help people with dementia. The potential of these technologies is clear, but what is so far uncertain is whether they are suitable in their existing commercial formats, how far they need to be purposefully designed for dementia or how far existing services are willing or able to integrate them into their service provision.

Alongside more general technologies, a number of apps have also been purposefully designed to assist people with dementia in making their home environments dementia friendly. Dementia-related apps have previously been designed for a range of activities, such as cognitive exercises, reminiscence or arts-based activities, rating places according to their dementia friendliness, and finally in relation to dementia-friendly design (see Example 4.2).

Example 4.2 'Iridis' dementia design app

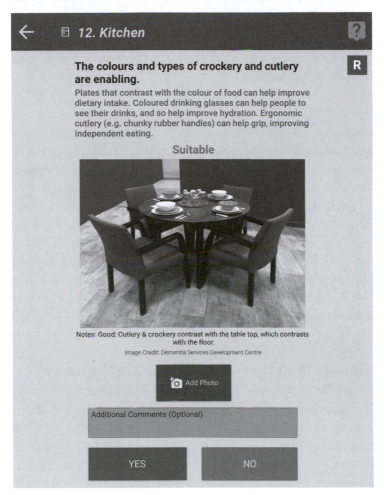

Figure 4.3 Screenshot of Iridis app

Iridis is a digital version of the Dementia Design Audit Tool developed at the Dementia Services Development Centre at the University of Stirling. Iridis takes the form of an app for smartphones or tablets, and enables individuals, family, health and social care professionals and others to conduct audits of physical spaces to ensure they are dementia friendly. Such physical spaces can include a residential care home, a public building or indeed a person's own home. The app provides guidance and recommendations about the layout and objects included within a physical space. Guidance can include recommendations in relation to flooring, wall coverings and colours, and suitability of furniture and furnishings, as well as suggesting changes to spaces to make them more suitable for people with dementia.

Also emerging from university research, the MindMate app provides a range of activities for people with dementia, including physical and mental exercises, information regarding nutrition and reminiscence activities.[5] A small-scale evaluation of MindMate found that the app was feasible as an intervention for people with dementia, and was effective when compared to practice as usual; however, larger studies are required in order to test its efficacy (McGoldrick 2017). Such technologies have a great deal of potential in enhancing the lives of people with dementia, but only if we are able to recognise how they are best integrated into people's lives, and only if we develop systems and services which can support their usage.

Challenges to the use of technology in the home

There are also numerous challenges which affect how far technologies can be integrated into dementia care practice. One of the most commonly experienced challenges is a lack of information about available technologies (Newton *et al.* 2016). A Scottish project called Dementia Circle, hosted by Alzheimer's Scotland, attempts to overcome this problem by crowdsourcing information from older people living with dementia and their carers living in Scotland about their experiences of using everyday technologies.[6] A similar UK project, called AT Dementia,[7] provides an information platform for assistive technologies, which is used as an information resource by people with dementia as well as other stakeholders including health and social care professionals (Burrow and Brooks 2012). Such information repositories have an important role that should be extended (Mieland *et al.* 2017). However, a lack of knowledge about information repositories such

---

5   www.mindmate-app.com
6   www.dementiacircle.org
7   www.atdementia.org.uk

as AT Dementia can limit the information health and social care professionals can provide (Newton *et al.* 2016). In addition, short-term funding models can often mean that becoming established and keeping up to date with technological advances over the longer term poses a challenge for the maintenance and updating of online resources.

Interoperability between devices and systems also poses an important problem. At present, many telecare and smart home technologies possess their own proprietary formats, forming 'walled gardens' which prevent usability between different device ecosystems (Greenhalgh *et al.* 2015). Such platforms may limit an individual's choice over technologies, but will have much greater implications for local authorities or health/social care organisations. These issues may limit the growth of smart home technologies by limiting the integration between different technologies and by reducing consumer choice. A number of third-party household devices are beginning to integrate Amazon's Alexa voice controls into their functionality, suggesting that interoperability between these platforms is possible, although it may require interventions at the level of public policy, such as standards frameworks, in order to drive interoperability between devices (Fisk 2015).

In addition, while many technologies have the potential to be used by people with dementia, they may not necessarily be suitable for people with dementia in their current forms. For example, despite being widely used within social care services, people with dementia frequently find the disembodied voices attached to existing community alarm and telecare systems frightening or confusing, a factor which often leads to their abandonment (Gibson *et al.* 2016; Greenhalgh *et al.* 2017; Orpwood *et al.* 2005). This means that there are unlikely to be universal solutions suitable for all people with dementia, and instead technologies must be used sensitively, based on the individual and personalised according to their needs. Such usage may require fundamentally different models of telecare service delivery than those offered at present (Greenhalgh *et al.* 2012).

Conclusion: home and the person-centred use of technology

The dominant way of using assistive technology at home is in the provision of care from a distance using telecare-based technologies. The dominance of telecare provided through health and social care agencies has currently focused and defined the assistive technology market, and has meant that technologies have prioritised managing the risks that living at home can bring for people with dementia, neglecting their potential in enabling people with dementia to participate in society (Bartlett and O'Connor 2010; Mort *et al.* 2013). There is scope for technology to do so much more than just managing risk. A mixed economy of technology, which includes both assistive technologies provided by care services and the wide range of everyday, commercially available technologies, can promote social participation, enjoyable activities and citizenship, and ultimately give people with dementia the opportunity to live a more engaged and engaging life (Astell *et al.* 2014b; Bowes and McColgan 2013).

A key determinant of whether technology is successfully adopted is how well technologies can fit into the personal, social and material contexts of the home. Understanding these contexts is fundamental to the successful deployment of technology; however, the technology or the services providing them frequently do not pay sufficient attention to these contexts when delivering technology-enabled care (Greenhalgh *et al.* 2013). The insensitive use of technology, either by individuals or by services, can make the home an isolated and isolating space, for example if care by people is replaced by care by machines, or if care is delivered in ways that restrict or even frighten the person in receipt of them (Mort *et al.* 2015; Oldman 2003; Percival and Hanson 2006). Technologies are re-making what we understand as care in both positive and negative ways, but this depends not on the technology per se, but in the ways in which designers, organisations and individuals decide how technologies should be used (Mort *et al.* 2015). As technologies continue to be put forward as a means to address the challenges posed by dementia care, questions about what constitutes the 'proper' use of technology, and whether the forms, structures and practices of care that emerge from these technologies are appropriate to people's needs, should continue to be asked. As a starting place for these conceptualisations, if we consider the use of technology in the home as situated within the individual, contextual arrangements of a person's lived life, we can develop technology solutions that will enable more people to live well with dementia.

Take-home points

* Enabling people to live at home is a key policy issue for health and social care agencies worldwide, with technology frequently being put forward as a means to enable people with dementia to age in place.

* A mixed economy of technologies for care is emerging that includes both assistive and everyday technologies, which are provided by both public bodies and private companies. This mixed economy is likely to grow in the future as the number of older people who are familiar and comfortable with technologies grows.

* Telecare, or systems of sensors able to monitor a person's activities in the home and manage the risks they may pose, is by far the most common form of assistive technology in dementia. However, technology also has the scope to enable people with dementia to continue with household activities, hobbies and interests, and keep in touch with friends and family.

* For technologies to make a positive difference to a person's life, they need to be introduced sensitively, according to that person's individual needs. A 'one size fits all' approach to technology in dementia does not work.

* When introducing technology, we should consider the 'little arrangements' a person has in the home that support the person, and introduce technologies based on these arrangements.

* Future general technologies such as smartphones and smart homes, alongside apps, have the potential to make significant contributions to dementia care in the home in the near future, but again should be used sensitively according to a person's preferences and needs.

Chapter 5

Outdoor Life and Technology with Dementia

Dr Rens Brankaert, *Assistant Professor,*
Eindhoven University of Technology, the Netherlands

Sandra Suijkerbuijk, *Researcher,*
Vilans and Eindhoven University of Technology, the Netherlands

Introduction

The ability to move around outdoors is important for all of us, but especially for people with dementia. It enhances independent living, allows them to be part of the community, and enables them to participate in social activities. Outdoor physical activity, particularly walking, plays an essential role in older adults' functional independence, whether they have cognitive challenges or not (Simonsick *et al.* 2005). To emphasise the importance of continuing activity outside the home, Silverstein and Parker (2002) argue that the quality of life of older people increases significantly with their ability to move around in their local outdoor environment. In addition, the ability to move freely outdoors has the potential to enhance self-esteem and independence.

In this chapter we examine the challenges people with dementia face when outside of their homes, and discuss technologies that have been developed to address these challenges. We cover these topics from both a design and a research perspective. In this way, we hope to enable those living, working and performing research in this field to find useful applications. In addition, we provide a new perspective on person-centred design, which we consider to be essential when aiming to provide suitable localisation, wayfinding and navigation technologies for people with dementia. This approach could also be implemented in the other domains described in this book or elsewhere.

The 'out of home' environment has two dimensions. The first relates to travel and navigation. This involves facilitating independent roaming outdoors and providing transport for people with dementia. Global Positioning System (GPS) localisation technologies designed to track and trace people with dementia also fall under this category. The second dimension covers developments in the public domain: how communities raise awareness, interact and communicate with people with dementia, for example training sessions for social contact or customer experience for people with dementia in shops, stores or museums, as part of the ongoing development of dementia-friendly communities in various countries (Crampton and Eley 2013; de Vugt and Dröes 2017; Phillipson et al. 2018). In this chapter, we mainly focus on the first dimension, travel and navigation, with relevant input for the second dimension.

Challenges related to navigation and wayfinding can arise for people with dementia. The severity of these challenges often correlates with the phase of the condition. The main issues are spatial orientation, memory and perception. Wayfinding refers to the way people mentally represent their environment and their ability to situate themselves physically within this space (Passini et al. 1998). People with dementia struggle to recall learn routes or landmarks, orientate or remember a location (Cushman, Stein and Duffy 2008). Deficits in perceiving and selecting relevant information from the environment make wayfinding difficult. In the early stages they might only get lost in unfamiliar places; however, as the disease progresses, they also tend to get lost in well-known places (Passini et al. 1998). Sheehan, Burton and Mitchell (2006) have suggested that traditional wayfinding solutions, such as visual notifications and public signs, can help people with dementia navigate. However, Passini et al. (1998) also showed that people with dementia are often confused by conventional wayfinding methods. This indicates that we should explore new options, and we feel that technology can play a major role here.

Recent developments in wayfinding technology

As already mentioned, wayfinding is a complex process for people with dementia, as both behavioural and cognitive actions are required (Passini et al. 1995). Even in familiar areas, people with dementia can face difficulties in finding their way, since they notice fewer landmarks and road signs (Uc *et al.* 2004). There are several ways in which we can support and protect people with dementia in navigation and wayfinding. A passive solution that can be used by caregivers for support is the ability to localise someone by tracking their location using GPS technology. In addition, people with dementia could carry a navigation aid to help them find the way during a walking trip. Furthermore, there are also possibilities to enhance the local outside context of people with dementia, using environmental and/or social design solutions.

GPS localisation

The market for GPS trackers is growing, as they are increasingly used to localise people with dementia, both in intramural and extramural care settings. People with dementia who go out and tend to face difficulties in wayfinding can use a passive version in the form of a tag (or in the earlier phases they can use a smartphone application). Family members or other caregivers can set up these devices to notify pre-programmed telephone numbers or email addresses if someone leaves a certain area or when someone pushes an emergency button. Systems developed for more advanced stages of dementia are non-interactive and usually only track people. Some are even designed in a way that the device cannot easily be detached (e.g. a wristband), although this can cause discomfort for the wearer. The prices of such systems can range from 70 to 1000 euros in the Netherlands (80–1200 USD and 60–880 GBP). These costs usually depend on the design of the system and extra services provided (Lukkien, Suijkerbuijk and Leeuw 2015).

The use of GPS trackers in the intramural care setting has become more popular in recent years (Lukkien *et al.* 2015). For example, the Dutch government is changing its policy for promoting greater autonomy and self-determination of people with dementia. In line with this, they promote respect for individuals as well as support that enables individuals to maintain control over their lives for as long as possible. Large national improvement programmes focus on delivering more person-centred care (Clarke, Hanson and Ross 2003) and, to enable this, there are, for example, investments in options that give more freedom to people with dementia. One promising example can be found at the care organisation Tante Louise in Bergen op Zoom, the Netherlands. They have an intramural care setting with radio-frequency identification (RFID) and GPS tags that are used in order to give every individual the freedom to walk around in the building, and even outside when possible. There is also a specially designed alert system that notifies neighbours when someone is lost in the area. Improved quality of care has been reported (Dierkx, Heshof and Remmerswaal 2017).

The GPS technology used to locate missing persons seems to be suitable for dementia care. However, as of today, most commercially available products lack one or more aspects that are important when designing products for people with dementia, such as price, accuracy and speed of operation, battery life, aesthetics, independent use and usability (Brankaert 2016; Hagethorn *et al.* 2008; Lukkien *et al.* 2015; McCabe and Innes 2013; Wan *et al.* 2016). In addition, the perspective of people with dementia tends to be neglected in the design of this type of technology, since their active interaction with the technology is not taken into account (Lazar, Edasis and Piper 2017). Although they need to carry the tracker with them when they go out, they do not understand what it is for.

Navigation devices

Navigation systems and applications, such as those contained in smartphones, can be used to enhance the wayfinding abilities of people with dementia. It is, however, important that these are easy to use for this target group. Challenges related to perceiving, selecting and processing relevant information from the environment make it more difficult for people with dementia to find their way (Lithfous, Dufour and Despres 2013). These deficits make it even more complicated to design an appropriate, safe and user-friendly navigation aid for them.

There are a range of universal navigation prompts that could be used to guide people to their destinations, for example, maps, text instructions, images and so on. The most frequently used are maps and text instructions. However, there is evidence that images can be of added value specifically for people with dementia (Goodman, Brewster and Gray 2005; Liu *et al.* 2008). For this user group, there is evidence that image prompting is preferred and it has been found to be more effective than audio prompting using vocal cues (Caffò *et al.* 2014; Liu *et al.* 2008). Nevertheless, there are situations in which images can cause confusion, such as when seasons change or when people look at a scene from a different viewpoint than in an image (Beeharee and Steed 2006). Enhancing wayfinding with landmark images can also be a valuable addition to pedestrian navigation systems for people with dementia.

Several small-scale experiments with newly designed navigation aids have been described by researchers (Hettinga *et al.* 2009; Holbø, Bøthun and Dahl 2013; Robinson *et al.* 2009). These indicate the potential of this type of technology for aiding people with dementia with wayfinding. As the design of the various systems differs, a common understanding is needed to improve the recognition, simplicity and ease of use of such technology.

Environmental and social design

In addition to the use of technology, there are also studies that focus more on environmental and social designs that can help people with dementia with wayfinding, both indoors and outdoors. In research on the environmental design of care institutions, designers often encourage people not to go outside at all. For example, Wan and colleagues (2016) describe constructional measures in care homes that include strategies such as heavy doors and camouflaged (or hidden) exits. Another commonly used measure is 'endless corridors'. This allows someone with dementia to take walks along a hallway which is in fact a circular route, so they never reach the exit. These types of solutions raise ethical questions, as they are designed to fool people with dementia. In addition, they conflict with person-centred approaches in design that encourage usability and improved quality of life (Brankaert 2016). These approaches have also received negative feedback from both formal and informal carers.

In the area of public service delivery, we see several trends emerging. Initiatives to create dementia-friendly communities can be found all over the world, in the UK, the Netherlands, Australia and more (Crampton and Eley 2013; de Vugt and Dröes 2017; Phillipson *et al.* 2018). In the Netherlands, this involves, for example, training clerks and shop assistants to identify people with dementia and interact appropriately with them. In York, UK, they focus on maintaining normalcy for people with dementia and involve them in decision-making processes (Crampton and Eley 2013). The main goal of these initiatives is to improve the way the public views dementia and to support people with dementia so that they can participate freely in the community despite having a cognitive disorder. Although such non-technological interventions are meaningful for the outdoor experience of people with dementia, the remainder of this chapter focuses on the application of technology in navigation and localisation systems.

Ethical considerations

GPS technology creates new opportunities that allow people with dementia to stay active outside their homes longer. Alongside the potential positive impact of these systems, electronic tracking also presents some ethical challenges. The use of GPS can result in infringement of privacy and human dignity when applied in the context of dementia (Astell 2006). Astell (2006) states that there is a lack of interventions designed to meet the individual needs and wishes of the target group. Furthermore, localisation technology might actually reduce contact between older people and other people in their social environment. While informal carers appear to be positive about the use of tracking technology, in the professional care environment its application seems to be disputed (Landau *et al.* 2010). The biggest differences are in the priority that informal caregivers give to the safety aspects of localisation technology, while formal caregivers focus more on privacy concerns related to tagging and tracking people.

Interestingly enough, privacy issues can differ among target groups and cultures. People with dementia participating in a study conducted by Lindsay and colleagues (2012) were not concerned about apparent reduced levels of privacy when using technology. They could not see why it would infringe their privacy, since their caregivers already have ways of knowing their whereabouts. The people with dementia were even comforted by such localisation systems because they would make their caregivers less worried. However, when people do not understand the functionality of such devices, they might get confused and fearful due to loss of control.

A design-led approach

As the example of the research by Lindsay and colleagues showed, it is very important to involve users in developing technology for people with dementia. Rather than taking a purely technology-driven approach, more suitable solutions can be found if we take a sensitive and inclusive approach to those we create technology for (Thompson Klein 2004). Design allows for such an approach. Designers are able to identify needs, conceptualise ideas, build prototypes, and take different perspectives into account (Krogstie 2012). Designers are able to deal with complex problems like dementia (Martin 2009), and integrate various, sometimes seemingly disparate, perspectives in a single concept. In addition, design research prescribes methods such as co-design (Sanders and Stappers 2008) and participatory design (Muller 2003; Robertson and Simonsen 2013) to make the target group(s) part of the design process itself. Dementia is such a distinct condition that these types of involvement are needed to ensure that technologies meet the needs of people with dementia directly (Branco, Quental and Ribeiro 2015; Brankaert and den Ouden 2017; Hendriks *et al.* 2014; Lindsay *et al.* 2012; Wallace *et al.* 2013). The involvement of and consultation with people with dementia is of particular importance in the quest for usable navigation and localisation applications due to dilemmas in the general ethical debate about tracking and tagging them.

In addition, research shows that existing GPS technology sometimes lacks design that takes usability and user experience into account. Robinson and colleagues (2009) concluded in their literature review that there are several problems with this technology, such as cost, the need for training and support, technical problems, the size of equipment, battery issues and increased demands on carers. Similar results were found in a Dutch study by care organisation Vilans (Lukkien *et al.* 2015), which also reported issues with the size of the device, the aesthetic appearance of devices, inaccuracy and problems with battery life. Since design for people with dementia can be challenging, it is important to include specific participatory approaches in a design process. To demonstrate different possible approaches and related results, we present three case studies related to navigation and wayfinding technology.

Case studies on the development of navigational aids

In the following case studies, different views on and approaches to the development of navigational aids are discussed. The first case shows the result of a more traditional product development process. The second case illustrates how this product is further developed in a more iterative and inclusive design process. The third and final case reveals a more design-driven approach to developing navigational aids for people with dementia. These three case studies show how different approaches result in different end products that can be used to help people with dementia with wayfinding.

Case study 5.1 Happy Walker

Happy Walker is an intervention developed in an Active Assisted Living (AAL) project (Suijkerbuijk *et al.* 2016). Extensive user research within this project showed an apparent need for navigation support for people with dementia in combination with various types of functionality such as planning tasks (Verhoeven *et al.* 2016). The Happy Walker system designed in the project offered multiple functionalities: to plan activities (see Figure 5.1), to travel and to memorize these activities. This application ran on a regular Android smartphone and was designed both for older adults in general and for people with dementia.

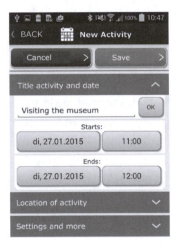

Figure 5.1 Planning screen in the Happy Walker V1 interface

Because the project focused on two user groups, the Happy Walker project led to a solution that failed to meet the needs of either of these user groups. The older adults mostly did not see the added value of some of the specifically designed services in the system. For example, they explained that they preferred to use their regular applications for keeping their agendas. The older adults felt a bit offended by the idea that they needed special guidance in planning activities, which was obviously designed for people with cognitive impairments. On the other hand, the people with dementia were confused by all the different options that the system offered. Usability tests revealed that people with dementia faced several problems when using the interface of the Happy Walker prototype shown in Figure 5.1 (Suijkerbuijk *et al.* 2016). By attempting to create an inclusive design that would serve multiple purposes, design-for-all resulted effectively in design for none.

Nevertheless, in this project, various insights were gained into the need for a navigation aid for people with dementia. The project team decided to further develop parts of the Happy Walker system in the Happy Walker 2.0 project.

Case study 5.2 Happy Walker 2.0

Various design research methods were used in order to first get a rich understanding of the needs of people with dementia and their informal caregivers (see Figure 5.2). The process started with paper prototype sessions with eight individuals with dementia and six informal caregivers. Insights from this exploratory process revealed the most important interface aspects, both from the perspective of someone with dementia and that of their informal caregiver. There were slight differences between these two perspectives, for example in relation to the clear presence of an emergency button, which was felt to be less important by those with dementia. One of the more remarkable design ideas provided by one of the participants was clarification of the starting point of the journey and the destination. This person with dementia designed an interface that always had a starting location at the bottom of the screen and an end location at the top. 'This makes it clear to me that I am going from point A to point B,' he said.

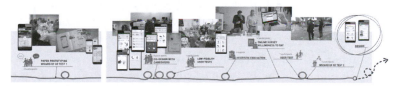

Figure 5.2 Design process of the Happy Walker 2.0

Using a co-design approach, we arrived at new insights and divergent perspectives to include in a new design proposal (see Figure 5.3). To evaluate the new concepts, we conducted two Wizard of Oz evaluation tests during the Happy Walker 2.0 design process. Wizard of Oz is a rapid-prototyping method for systems that are costly to build or require new technology (Wilson and Rosenberg 1988). In this method, a human simulates the system's intelligence and interacts with the participant through a real or mock-up computer interface.

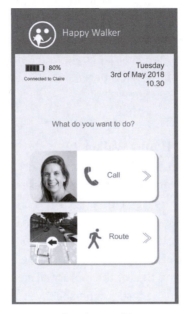

Figure 5.3 New interface design of the Happy Walker 2.0

The first Wizard of Oz test with Happy Walker 2.0 included a set of screenshots of a route that the researcher and the participant had to subsequently walk along. All participants were asked to walk a short pre-defined route in their own neighbourhood. Since the researcher visited every participant in their own home, some preparation was needed. Happy Walker used Google Street View pictures, therefore the researchers had to digitally 'walk' the route before the test in Google Maps for every participant to record the route. This test helped the researchers get insights into whether the different screens were understandable for the people with dementia and if they were able to navigate with the information provided. The same eight participants from the paper prototype sessions took part in this study.

In a later phase of the project, when the application was working properly, we focused on understanding audio prompts. Again, before implementing such functionality, we did another Wizard of Oz test with three new participants. One researcher had a Bluetooth speaker in his bag and operated a smartphone with pre-programmed voice prompts (e.g. 'Turn left at the next intersection'). Participants responded well to the audio prompts. Results showed that the audio prompts were not crucial to the usability of the system. They served only as an extra cue because participants were already able to navigate with only visual cues; therefore it was decided to postpone the further development and implementation of the audio prompts.

Both Wizard of Oz user tests provided many useful insights into usability and the experience of the individuals with dementia, without the need to actually build in the functionalities. In both tests we found this to be a valuable research method for people with dementia, since they do not need to imagine how something would work for them and the feedback on the system can be obtained directly, avoiding reflections afterwards, which might be difficult for people with cognitive decline (Orpwood *et al.* 2007; Suijkerbuijk *et al.* 2015).

Throughout the project, a married couple were consulted at several points in time. The researchers visited the man (who had dementia) and the woman at their home and at their convenience. By giving them a voice in the project, they steered the development of Happy Walker 2.0 throughout the process, including every aspect of the design. One useful insight came when the husband was confused by the word 'Back' in a back-button on the navigation screen. 'It is confusing because I think the system wants me to go back to the point where I walked from.' This shows that even in the later phases of development, it is crucial to get insights from people with dementia themselves in order to discover all the aspects of a concept that need modification. The perspective of the user can so easily be misunderstood.

The final design of the Happy Walker consists of two smartphone applications (Figure 5.4). One – with limited functionality – is designed to be operated by the person with dementia, and there are several functionalities which are optional and can be either turned on or off by the informal caregiver. Optional functionalities include the ability to navigate to several pre-programmed destinations and the ability to call several informal caregivers (rather than just one emergency contact). All settings can be handled by the smartphone application intended for the informal caregiver. By including a separate application, the number of screens in the application for the person with dementia could be vastly reduced in order to make the application usable for most people with dementia.

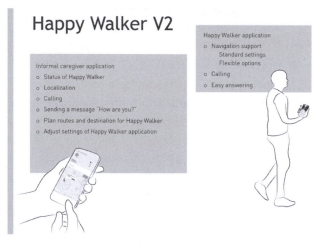

Figure 5.4 Explanation of the new Happy Walker 2.0 concept

Case study 5.3 Homing Compass

In this case study, we cover the design and field evaluation of the Homing Compass. This is a device that can be used to support people with dementia who wish to find their way home individually. The system was designed together with people with dementia as well as dementia experts. The idea was that the design should aid people with dementia directly. It should guide them home in a safe manner, free from anxiety. Also, the device should not look too technical, compared to, for example, a smartphone (Robinson *et al.* 2009). We therefore decided to use a recognisable metaphor for wayfinding: a compass. In addition, the appearance of a compass might suggest 'bringing you home'.

User involvement

For the first iteration, we involved six formal caregivers. Many different aesthetic prototypes of wayfinding devices were created, with buttons, screens, lights and sound effects, which could be mixed and matched. These were evaluated together with the formal caregivers using a co-design approach. We didn't want to involve people with dementia yet because this phase was still very conceptual. The design was generally well received, but often caution was expressed as to whether it would work for people with late-stage dementia. Other concerns related to people with dementia having difficulty learning new things. The main message was that the design had to be simple yet recognisable, and the learning curve had to be very short.

In a second iteration, we involved people with dementia and their caregivers to review a wayfinding compass that had been designed based on input from the caregivers. A small display was added to provide feedback about where the compass was pointing. We also added a central button, with a home icon. This button was included both to provide auditory feedback and to add a visual reference to 'home'. In total, four people with dementia and three informal caregivers participated. In the focus group, we used a schematic drawing and an interactive non-working prototype. In general, they responded positively to our design. However, there was a general desire for simplicity and extra buttons were seen as confusing. In terms of sturdiness it was remarked that the device should be both weather- and impact-proof, as the risk of accidents increases with dementia. In addition, most participants preferred a size that could fit in one's hand. Finally, the home icon we added was felt to be confusing: it suggested that the device was pointing away from home.

Based on this input a final design was proposed. The main functionality of the 'Homing Compass' is a simple navigation system that points homewards using a large arrow, supported by a indicative LED ring. Additional features such as a map, auditory feedback or help and alternative route selection were removed from the device to maintain its simplicity, as users and experts preferred this. The design's look and feel resembles that of an actual compass by using familiar materials such as wood and metal. The physical prototype is shown in Figure 5.5.

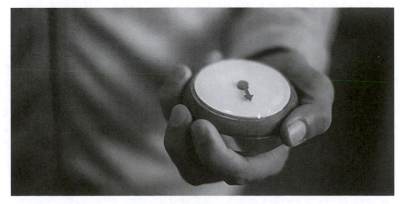

Figure 5.5 The Homing Compass

Field evaluation setup

To evaluate our design, we conducted field evaluations of the working prototype with end-users in a natural context (see Figure 5.6). The working prototype was functional in pointing people to a pre-destined location by use of an arrow and an LED ring. However, the GPS coordinates still had to be hard-coded into the device by the researchers. Eight couples participated, each consisting of an informal caregiver and a person with dementia. Each participant with dementia was in the early to mild stages of dementia. We designed a study that could be performed in about two hours, with a focus on using the device for navigational and wayfinding purposes. The study was set up as follows:

1. The person with dementia was instructed to use the Homing Compass from home to find a pre-set location in their neighbourhood (point A).

2. After reaching point A they were guided by the Homing Compass to a second location nearby that was slightly more difficult to reach (point B).

3. Finally, from this location they were pointed home by the Homing Compass.

For the comfort of the person with dementia the informal caregiver would walk alongside; however, they were instructed not to help. The researcher walked behind them as a non-participatory observer. The device pointed directly towards a location in a bird's eye view and therefore they still had to make their own decisions in dealing with roads and traffic. A semi-structured interview was then held at home afterwards, lasting approximately 30 minutes.

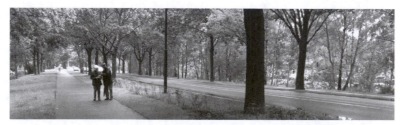

Figure 5.6 A couple walking in their neighbourhood during the evaluation test of the Homing Compass

Field evaluation results

We found that seven of the eight participants with dementia managed to successfully find their way home. Three participants were very positive about the design and expressed a desire to use it in the future. Two participants found the device too simple and reported no need for it yet. Two other participants felt it to be beneficial for them, and had additional comments about features they wished to add to the device before they were comfortable using it. Finally, one participant found it very difficult to use.

Discussion

In this chapter, we aimed to show the promise of technology for supporting people with dementia when outdoors. Although there is clear demand, since the policy in the Netherlands is to stimulate independent living, the actual uptake of wayfinding technology is still low. We argue that more person-centred solutions, as illustrated in Case studies 5.2 and 5.3, could change this, as they cater more persuasively to the needs of people with dementia. Therefore, to achieve such positive results in a design process, we need to embrace a different type of design approach that is person-centred and inclusive.

The growing demands that dementia is likely to place on formal and informal care in the near future have led to growing interest in how technology can ease this situation. However, technology is still often developed without involving people with dementia directly (Span *et al.* 2013; Topo 2009). Fortunately, there are more studies emerging that suggest and apply participatory design processes in the development of technology for people with dementia. However, many projects are still based on a technology push, where the technology drives value rather than people.

The first case study in this chapter is based on a project from the European Active Assisted Living joint programme. The aim of this programme is to provide equipment and services for the independent living of elderly people. The programme funds projects that consists of small and medium-sized enterprises (SMEs), research bodies and end-user organisations from 17 different countries (AAL Association n.d.). Unfortunately, many solutions created in the programme focus on technological development, at the expense of usability and the existence of a suitable (user-centred) design process. This was to some extent the case in the Happy Walker project. Most AAL solutions are technology-driven and they are not adequately centred on service innovations and social innovations (Depaoli 2016). Nevertheless, the projects in this programme are generating valuable knowledge for the development of new technical solutions for people with dementia. The second case study, for example, showed how a more focused project leads to an actual usable product. And, in the third case study, it is shown how a person-centred starting point leads to a person-centred technological design in line with the needs and wishes of people living with dementia.

Personhood in technology design

As highlighted by Newell and colleagues (2011), we see a lack of aesthetic and personal considerations in most products that are designed for older and disabled people. This might be evidence of the low engagement of companies with their actual target group, assuming that older and disabled people are uninterested in aesthetics, and, unlike other groups we design for, are motivated only by the functionality of products. We see this same problem of disengagement in the development of products for people with dementia as well. As those with dementia are often not properly understood, they are protected and treated as if they are considered to be ill, but by doing this we strip away their identity and personhood (Kontos 2005). We also ignore the evidence of the successes of more person-centred approaches (Treadaway and Kenning 2016). Similarly, in technology, we should deliberately design with a person-centred perspective, and use this to empower people with dementia (Lazar *et al.* 2017; Morrissey, McCarthy and Pantidi 2017). We should include the perspective of people with dementia such as experience, quality of life, wellbeing and fulfilment, instead of a focus on needs of carers such as efficiency, safety and organisation. Both the case studies Happy Walker 2.0 and the Homing Compass show how designers can use creative skills and methods to overcome these sometimes-conflicting perspectives in a balanced process (Brankaert, den Ouden and Brombacher 2015).

Our experience in the Happy Walker 2.0 project and with the Homing Compass is in line with research by Holbø, Bøthun and Dahl (2013), who identify a shift in conceptualising this type of technology for the outdoor life of people with dementia. Instead of a more surveillance-based model, Holbø and colleagues conclude from their co-design activities with people with dementia that outdoor technological interventions should be seen as tools that collaboratively take care of safety in an enjoyable and respectful way. We hope we have inspired you with this review and sketched a new direction for this exciting field of research and development for people living with dementia.

Take-home points

* There is an evident benefit for people with dementia to maintain their mobility for active outdoor activities.

* Technology can and should be used to develop new travel and navigational aids to overcome wayfinding challenges by people with dementia.

* Technological support systems for people with dementia should be designed in a participatory and inclusive way to increase usability and usefulness.

* Focus on a person-centred design approach, as illustrated in the Happy Walker 2.0 and Homing Compass cases, allows the empowerment of people with dementia in design.

Acknowledgements

We would like to express great appreciation towards the people with dementia, their caregivers and others involved to make the studies described possible. Additionally, we gratefully acknowledge the financial support from the European AAL Joint Programme, the Dutch funding agency ZonMw and Interreg NWE. In particular, the work here has been supported by the AAL Happy Walker project (AAL-2011-4-088) and the Innovate Dementia NWE Interreg project. The Homing Compass described in Case study 5.3 was realised in collaboration with Rian de Jong.

Chapter 6

Leisure Activities and Technology with Dementia

Dr Phil Joddrell, *Research Associate,*
Centre for Assistive Technology and Connected Healthcare,
University of Sheffield, UK

Dr Sarah Kate Smith, *Research Associate,*
Salford Institute of Dementia, University of Salford, UK

Introduction

Leisure is an enjoyable and meaningful way of passing the time, away from domestic chores, daily activities and paid work. What we view as leisure is subjective, in that it means different things to different people. Activities can be sedentary, such as completing a crossword or reading a book, or active, such as going for a walk or playing golf. Leisure activities are enjoyable because we get pleasure from doing them independently, for example knitting or completing a jigsaw puzzle, or with others, such as playing games or singing in a choir. Leisure activities can also be meaningful if they provide us with opportunities to use our skills and abilities, such as painting or playing a musical instrument. In this chapter our definition of leisure includes individual and group activities such as dancing, listening to or playing music, singing, gardening and other hobbies.

Interest in leisure activities does not go away when people have dementia. Indeed, there is a huge need for something enjoyable and rewarding to do during the day, particularly activities that are social or can be carried out independently. A recent scoping review (Hedman, Lindqvist and Nygård 2016) identified several factors important to people living with dementia in relation to activities that they want to keep doing. These include activities that convey social values and wellbeing through staying connected to friends; activities that support significant roles, such as being a good host or being a sociable person; activities that reduce demands on others to avoid being a burden; and activities that increase health and safety, such as getting around safely out of doors (Hedman *et al.* 2016). However, people with dementia may withdraw from previously enjoyed activities, especially group-based ones, through embarrassment at not being able to participate as they used to, or difficulty accessing them, for example because of a need to take public transport. The 2012 World Alzheimer's Report found that 40 per cent of people with dementia described feeling excluded from everyday life, with almost 60 per cent feeling avoided or having lost contact with family and friends (Batsch and Mittelman 2012).

To address these challenges, various initiatives have been developed offering a wide variety of leisure activities to people with dementia. The following brief list highlights the range of approaches and initiatives emerging to provide meaningful leisure activities for people with dementia. Some of the following examples are research projects, while others are community-based programmes that have not involved academic evaluation. However, all are looking at ways to engage people living with dementia in leisure pursuits.

Outdoor activities

Participation in outdoor activities has been shown to have a number of benefits for people with dementia. Examples include guided interactions with horses, which have been shown to have a positive impact on the physiology and behaviour of individuals with dementia (Dabelko-Schoeny *et al.* 2014). Berkshire-based Younger People with Dementia is a charity focused on people with dementia keeping busy by offering a large selection of activities including running, canoeing, walking, badminton, table tennis, furniture restoration, reading and gardening (Hussey 2016). The Sensory Trust organises walking groups for people with dementia and their carers to get outdoors and meet like-minded people. THRIVE, on the other hand, is an initiative developed in association with the University of Loughborough focusing on gardens and gardening for people living with dementia (Sempik, Aldridge and Becker 2002). Another example is Dementia Adventure, a UK-based charity connecting people with dementia with the outdoors and their community.

Community-based activities

Attending art galleries with trained guides can improve confidence and engagement for people with dementia (MacPherson *et al.* 2009), and art galleries have been described as 'a physically valued place that provides intellectual stimulation and offers opportunities for social inclusion' (Camic, Baker and Tischler 2016, p.1033). Another community activity is facilitated storytelling, which provides creative expression to positively impact quality of life (Phillips, Reid-Arndt and Pak 2010) and support conversation between people with dementia and caregivers (Fels and Astell 2011). Other community-based activities include Matinée, run by Arts Derbyshire, which organises 'dementia-friendly' cinema screenings across Derbyshire. Dementia cafés can also be found across the UK, providing community spaces for people with dementia and their carers to gather socially (Capus 2005). In Australia, the charity Dance Health Alliance is delivering movement programmes for people with a range of cognitive and physical challenges including dementia (Korebrits, Gajjarr and Palmer 2017). Singing for the Brain is another popular activity, widely accepted as having health and wellbeing benefits for people with dementia and their carers (Osman, Tischler and Schneider 2016).

Technology

As in other aspects of life, technology is increasingly being used to support people with dementia to participate in leisure activities. This includes digital versions of some of the activities mentioned above and again includes both group and individual activities. For example, House of Memories is a museum-led dementia awareness programme that offers a downloadable application ('app') for smartphones and tablet computers that can be used to explore historical artefacts (National Museums Liverpool 2012). As with House of Memories, many activities utilise off-the-shelf technologies popular with the general population. For example, Dove and Astell (2017c) reported cognitive, physical and social benefits through participation in a virtual bowling group for people with dementia, while Neubauer and colleagues (2018) tested virtual Tai Chi in participants' homes; both of these projects utilised the Microsoft Xbox Kinect system. Schikhof and Wauben (2016) found that virtual cycling using a commercially available product provided by a small Dutch company (Wiltraco) had a positive effect on mood and behaviour, especially when viewing personally relevant images while cycling.

Other studies have explored the potential of viewing art on a tablet (Tyack and Camic 2017), creating art on touchscreen devices (Leuty *et al.* 2013) and using interactive digital technologies to facilitate interactions with art or nature with people with dementia (Twedt, Proffitt and Hearn 2014). Digital storytelling delivered using an app provides a creative means for people to tell their own stories through vocalisations, images and music (Critten and Kucirkova 2017). CIRCA (Computer Interactive Reminiscence and Conversation Aid; Alm *et al.* 2004) is a multimedia touchscreen system that can support one-to-one conversations (Alm *et al.* 2009) and provides a cognitively stimulating group activity for people with dementia (Astell *et al.* 2018b). Building on this, the same researchers developed Living in the Moment (LIM), a suite of digital touchscreen games (Astell *et al.* 2014a), and also created and tested a prototype interactive touchscreen tool to promote musical creativity with people with dementia, which was found to be enjoyable and easy to use (Riley *et al.* 2009). This is unsurprising, as music is regarded as beneficial for people with dementia, in part because the areas of the brain responsible for encoding musical memory are relatively well preserved in Alzheimer's disease, and as such people show similar responses to both healthy young adults and age-matched controls (Jacobsen *et al.* 2015). Consequently, many projects and initiatives have been launched to provide music for people with dementia. For example, Playlist for Life is a UK music and dementia charity who offer a digital music service through the Spotify catalogue to collate the music of a person's life, keeping them connected to themselves and their loved ones throughout their dementia journey. However, a 2017 review of the way music is used in dementia care concluded that the use of pre-recorded music is not always positive, and that 'further clarification of protocols for music use and closer investigation of variables that influence individual response to music' is required (Garrido *et al.* 2017, p.1129).

Touchscreen tablet computers

As demonstrated above, off-the-shelf technologies such as touchscreen tablet computers offer the potential to promote enjoyable activity with people with varying levels of cognitive impairment. This is because they are flexible and can be personalised to an individual or group.

Exploring the potential of touchscreen technologies to provide leisure opportunities for people living with dementia is a central focus of our own research (Astell *et al.* 2010, 2016; Joddrell, Hernandez and Astell 2016; Smith and Mountain 2012). A recent review identified the variety of ways in which touchscreen devices, including tablet computers, have been utilised with people living with dementia (Joddrell and Astell 2016). Touchscreens are favoured because the format reduces the demand of hand–eye coordination that is required when using a desktop computer with a mouse and cursor (Wandke, Sengpiel and Sönksen 2012), making it a more effective control method for people with dementia.

Anecdotally, we are hearing more and more that care providers, both professional and informal, are buying tablet computers for use with people living with dementia. Out of the box, however, these devices have very little to offer beyond basic tasks such as Internet browsing, email management and word processing, as so much of their functionality is reliant on downloadable apps, some of which we have mentioned above. Consequently, the extent to which a tablet computer can be considered useful and suitable is defined by its apps. Not only do new users require practical information such as how to acquire them, connect them to the Internet and set up an account, they also need to consider which apps they should download in order to use the tablet computer most effectively.

Case studies

Focusing on existing apps (as opposed to developing new software), we present two case studies: the first describing how touchscreen computers can promote enjoyment in both group and individual sessions, and with people living with dementia both at home and attending care services; and the second looking at how collaborations between users, researchers and developers have led to the development of a tool to help people find suitable apps.

Case study 6.1 Practicalities of using tablets for leisure

This work was conducted as part of a doctoral research programme exploring the potential of touchscreen tablet computers to address the challenge of people with dementia lacking enjoyable things to do in their day-to-day lives. The importance of personalising technologies with people experiencing varying levels of dementia was examined, in two different settings: a social group attending a day service, and one-to-one in people's homes (Smith 2015).

Group setting

Those attending the day service had been living with a diagnosis of dementia for some time. Some lived alone while others were managing to maintain their independence with the help of family members. The aims of the group are to provide people with moderate levels of dementia living at home with opportunities to improve wellbeing, develop friendships and maintain existing skills. The researcher became a volunteer at the group prior to the research starting in order to get to know members, staff and volunteers, and to observe 'usual' activities enjoyed during group sessions. The overall aim of the research was to explore the potential of off-the-shelf technology in promoting enjoyable activities with people with dementia. The 'usual' activities enjoyed in this day service consisted of traditional games of dominoes and solitaire, use of physical life story albums and reference books, and jigsaws and other puzzles. The researcher was keen to use these familiar activities as apps on the tablet computers as well as additional, more novel activities that would be new to group members. These included interactive, sensory apps like the 'Virtual Fish Pond' and 'Fireworks'. Standard apps already installed on the tablet computers were also hugely popular, including the built-in camera for taking and having fun with photographs, or FaceTime for making video calls between small groups. Sessions using the tablet computers took place once a week for a period of four weeks. Each session lasted approximately one hour and always took place before lunchtime. Four tablet computers were used simultaneously within small groups of three to four people, who were seated around a large table within one overall group of up to 20. All of the research sessions were video recorded, allowing for in-depth analysis of verbal and non-verbal behaviour of the members during engagement with the tablet computers.

The quantity of apps downloaded onto the tablet computers increased as the researcher got to know the group better. Initially, around 12 apps were downloaded by the researcher based on observations of the group enjoying familiar or usual activities. If someone mentioned, for example, their love of playing the guitar, piano or drums then the researcher would search for and download apps that enabled this, either during the same session or ready for the next one. The flexibility of the tablets and the plethora of available apps enabled the personalisation of the devices to the voiced preferences of the group.

When the research began it was apparent very quickly how both personal choices and individual differences play a part when engaging with leisure activities. For example, some groups enjoyed engaging with competitive turn-taking activities such as Memory Match or Hangman, that got increasingly more difficult as the levels progressed. In contrast, others preferred activities that were more light-hearted – for example, Talking Tom – allowing for laughter, joking and fun (see Figure 6.1).

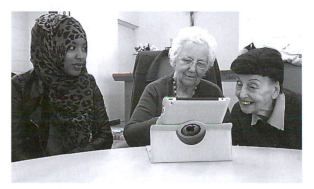

Figure 6.1 Touchscreen tablet computer activities in a group setting

Overall, participants in the group setting engaged with leisure activities and with each other through the medium of technology. Personalising the devices to the groups' expressed wishes was appropriate as there was enjoyment in the experience of taking part in familiar activities that had been effectively recreated for the touchscreen format. Possibly the most popular of these familiar activities were the jigsaw puzzles, although there was also enjoyment evident during participation with the sensory apps, with people gasping in wonder at how clever the tablet computers were during use of the Fireworks app. The groups were keen to try these novel activities and the majority were very capable of interacting with the tablet computers, provided that appropriate support was in place. This was an exploratory study, so no formal measures were taken of cognition, health or quality of life.

One-to-one settings

In parallel with the group sessions, a second study was undertaken involving people living at home who had received a recent diagnosis of dementia. In-depth interviews were conducted to find out hobbies and activities that were important to each individual, including some they felt they could no longer engage with due to their changing circumstances. Tablets were personalised based on the information and knowledge gained through these interviews. None of the participants in this phase of the research were attending community groups or other social events, either through choice or lack of opportunity.

As with the group study, all technology sessions were video recorded for the purposes of data analysis. Sessions took place once a week for four weeks and the participants did not need prompting or reminding of their last session. Indeed, they were more likely to be waiting at the window or on the doorstep when the researcher arrived. The tablets were personalised before the first session took place. In response to their preferences, the extensive list of apps included football, dress making, cooking, coin collecting, family trees and archaeology.

As in the group study, participants' individual differences were clear and defined. For some, the research became their own weekly technology session, and participants would create 'wish lists' between sessions of all the activities they were keen to engage with based on past or present interests. For others, the research sessions were more social and an excuse to enjoy some company, a cup of tea and a biscuit. In this sense, the apps on the devices tended to support social contact, interactions and conversations, for example listening to music or watching videos on YouTube. However, all activities were freely chosen by each participant because they were meaningful and had purpose, resulting in a greater chance of meeting the individual's needs and requirements.

Overall, the participants using tablet computers at home positively welcomed the opportunities that this study offered. For some, this meant increasing their social interactions; for others, increasing their knowledge and experience of both new and existing hobbies and interests. This project confirmed the appropriateness of personalised technologies that are tailored to the individual. Personalising technologies and providing choice was of paramount importance to the success of the devices being positively received by the majority. In the history of dementia interventions, there has been a tendency to generalise peoples' experiences, that is, to regard them as all the same (Bartlett and O'Connor 2007). Thus, if one person with dementia has difficulties using tablet computers, it might be assumed that the whole population of people with dementia will have the same difficulty. However, there is growing evidence challenging this view and of how technology can extend retained capabilities despite dementia (Astell *et al.* 2014a). It has often been reported that people living with dementia lack in opportunities to engage with technologies, but rarely do they lack in desire to do so (Nygård 2008).

This first case study demonstrates the potential in personalising tablet computers for people with dementia with apps that are of particular interest to them, in order to facilitate engaging leisure activities. This study highlighted the role of a skilled supporter to personalise the technology, and the need for time, resources and expertise to successfully utilise tablet computers and apps. This presents a significant challenge for families, professionals and users themselves to find the apps they are looking for within the huge quantity available. Furthermore, once apps have been accessed, there are no guarantees that they will be appropriate for the group or individual living with dementia. In order for these exciting and rewarding opportunities to become more widely achievable, a simplified process is required for finding apps that are suitable for people with dementia.

Case study 6.2 AcTo Dementia

The problem of app selection is easily demonstrated. When the first case study started in 2011, the number of apps available in the Apple iTunes App Store was 166,000. In 2017, this figure had risen to 2.3 million (Statista 2017). Therefore, finding apps that meet any user's requirements is a challenge, but where those requirements are more complex, as with dementia, the challenge becomes even greater.

We started the AcTo Dementia (Accessible Touchscreen apps for Dementia) project to address this challenge through four key objectives:

- Identifying features within existing touchscreen apps that increase their accessibility for people living with dementia.

- Developing an evidence-based, publicly available app selection framework supporting people to find touchscreen apps that are the most accessible examples of their type.

113

- Collaborating with app developers to improve the accessibility of existing apps for people living with dementia.

- Creating a website that publishes recommendations for accessible apps for people with dementia, as well as offering support guides and a community forum.

To achieve these aims, we recruited 66 people living with dementia to participate in testing touchscreen apps across three separate studies. In contrast to the first case study, this research explored the potential of people with dementia using touchscreen tablets independently (i.e. without the presence of a supporter). Our participants all lived in care services, and prior to working with us had limited experience with modern off-the-shelf technology (exemplified by the fact that none had ever used a touchscreen tablet computer before). Despite this, the vast majority were able to play the touchscreen games independently, with varying levels of progression but consistently high levels of reported enjoyment (Astell *et al.* 2016). For each gameplay session, we set up the environment to maximise the potential for independence by using video cameras to record the experience of the participants and their interactions with the app, thereby allowing the researcher to retreat out of sight (see Figure 6.2). After each session, the researcher conducted a short questionnaire with the participant to collect feedback about their experience. This method was used to allow each participant to contribute data both verbally and practically.

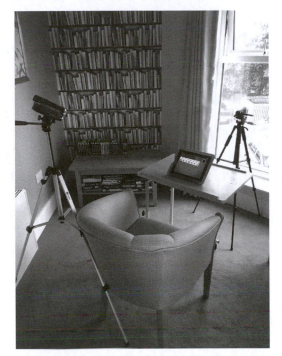

Figure 6.2 An example of how the equipment was set up within a care setting for data collection sessions in the AcTo Dementia project

The video recordings of each gameplay session were viewed by the researcher using the Observer™ video analysis software, through which every participant interaction with the app was coded (see Figure 6.3). This allowed us to see which features of the apps were facilitating successful interactions and which features were contributing to unsuccessful interactions. Several barriers to independent gameplay were identified with regard to the accessibility of the apps and the specific requirements of people with dementia. These included confusion between two different methods of touchscreen control ('tap' and 'drag-and-drop'), the distracting presence of menu bars or option buttons and a prompt feature that was not often used. These barriers were discussed with the developers of the two apps, and design adaptations were agreed collaboratively in an attempt to improve their accessibility for people living with dementia. This approach demonstrates the role of the researcher as a go-between to ensure that the complex needs of people with dementia can be communicated to an industry that would otherwise be unlikely to seek their input.

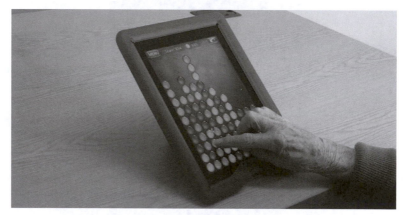

Figure 6.3 A participant in the AcTo Dementia project playing the puzzle game Bubble Explode independently

Using this information, and the findings from our literature review (Joddrell and Astell 2016), we created an app selection tool by compiling a checklist of accessibility features that contribute to the successful design of touchscreen apps for people living with dementia (Joddrell *et al.* 2016). This tool has since been used to identify many more apps that are published on our project website,[1] forming a catalogue of apps that have an increased chance of being accessible for people with dementia. By featuring as wide a range of apps as possible, we can help to facilitate the personalisation of touchscreen devices. The website also has a forum where people can share experiences of using the apps we recommend, or other ones they have found successful, as well as suggesting games and other activities they would like us to search for and evaluate.

In addition to our work with research participants, we have also sought the input of people living with dementia as expert advisers throughout the AcTo Dementia project. This has been, and will continue to be, an essential part of our process of investigating the accessibility requirements of touchscreen apps for dementia. The project commenced with a visit to the South Yorkshire Dementia Research Advisory Group at the point when we had some preliminary ideas for the first study. A later visit to the group was arranged when the AcTo

1   www.actodementia.com

Dementia project name and website were being discussed, and the group members provided helpful input in finalising the name and design. Finally, during a visit to the Alzheimer's Association International Conference in Toronto, Canada, in 2016, we were able to arrange several visits to local Alzheimer's Society groups to gather feedback on the fully functional website and some of the more recently recommended apps.

We feel strongly that our research has been strengthened with regular input from people living with dementia as the intended users of both the website and apps. Their involvement has delivered a range of impacts, from minor amendments to larger-scale changes, for example, the decision to include the word 'dementia' in the AcTo name. Originally, in an attempt to minimise the potential for stigmatisation, we opted not to have the term 'dementia' in our name. However, in discussions with the research advisory group members, it was pointed out that without the inclusion of the word 'dementia', people with the condition would not recognise that any linked resources were of benefit to them. This example is evidence that sometimes we can over-complicate matters as researchers, as well as further demonstrating the importance of involving people living with the condition in our decisions.

By involving people with dementia regularly during the course of our project, we have been able to stay focused on their needs. We believe this project demonstrates ways in which people with dementia can contribute to app development and evaluation. We have also highlighted how researchers can act as intermediaries between user groups with complex needs and those in the creative industry, identifying methods of collecting information and working collaboratively to implement change. Furthermore, as a counter-argument to so much of the stigma surrounding dementia, we would like to highlight that as a result of a strong and sustained input from people living with dementia, two leading apps in the world's most popular app stores now contain dementia accessibility features; and these apps are not specialist 'dementia versions' but are the same apps that everybody else has access to.

The stigma attached to the term 'dementia' has an impact on everyone affected by the condition, but most markedly upon those people living with a diagnosis (Batsch and Mittelman 2012). While media representation very often facilitates this stigma, it is by no means the only responsible agency; in reality this responsibility is shared much more systemically within our care systems (Benbow and Jolley 2012). While the overt message of the AcTo Dementia project is one of how collaborative working can lead to the increased access of leisure activities through everyday technologies, there is also an underlying message that seeks to challenge the myths and preconceptions that exist about what people living with a dementia diagnosis can and cannot do.

Future developments

In this chapter, we have used the example of tablet computers to illustrate how people living with dementia can access leisure activities. In the first example, personalisation of the devices was achieved through close collaboration with a researcher, where the existing interests and hobbies of each user were discussed, and apps were downloaded to match these interests. In the second example, a process was initiated to identify and share existing leisure apps that are the most accessible for people living with dementia. In each of these examples, the majority of participants were not existing users of technology, and the devices (i.e. tablet computers) were being introduced to people for the first time. Now and in the future, increasing numbers of people who receive a diagnosis of dementia will be more familiar with tablet computers and other everyday technologies associated with leisure activities (such as smartphones, video games consoles, etc.). Therefore, the questions that researchers, clinicians and developers will need to address will start to shift. For example, at the moment we are interested in investigating the accessibility of leisure apps so that we can introduce new opportunities for people living with dementia. In ten years' time, this information will be valuable as it will allow people who are existing app users to continue to enjoy the leisure activities with which they are familiar. This has the potential to prevent the development of a 'digital divide', where people diagnosed with dementia are excluded from a digital world that provides such a wide range of leisure opportunities.

It is also inevitable that what we now consider to be everyday technologies will also evolve, and emerging technology is already starting to be used for the purpose of leisure both in the general population and with people with dementia. Examples include virtual and augmented reality (Moyle *et al.* 2017) and robotics (Abdollahi *et al.* 2017). With all new technologies there is an element of the unknown relating to adoption and longevity, but in principle anything that has the potential to provide leisure activity opportunities should be considered for use by people living with dementia to avoid the aforementioned 'digital divide' from developing. It is hoped that what has already been discovered through the extensive research into leisure activities and technology for people with dementia can at least be used as a guide as to how we can approach the use of emerging technologies in the same context.

Take-home points

* A diagnosis of dementia should not limit the choice of leisure activity people are offered.

* Maintaining previous activities, hobbies and roles is important to people with dementia.

* In addition, people may benefit from being offered engaging ways to try new things.

* Sometimes dementia can impair a person's ability to communicate what leisure activities they would enjoy doing, but it should not be assumed that this is indicative that they are unable or unwilling to participate.

* People with dementia may need encouragement and support to continue engaging with leisure activities.

* Activities enjoyed in leisure time can be more meaningful after a diagnosis of dementia as they help to keep minds active and can emphasise all the things that the person does well.

Acknowledgements

We are very grateful to the managers, staff and service users of Darnall Dementia Group (Darnall Dementia Trust), Midhurst Road, Cotleigh, Springwood, Knowle Hill, Hawkhills (Sheffcare), Park View (Sanctuary Care), Prior Bank, Herries Lodge (Anchor), Abbey Grange (Country Court Care), Walkley Lodge (Roseberry Care) and Loxley Park (Signature), without whom the research described in the case studies would not have been possible.

Chapter 7

Technology Use by People with Dementia

Ken Clasper, Tom *and* Maureen Hawkins, Ann Johnson *and* Keith Oliver, *with* Nada Savitch, *Independent Consultant, London, UK*

This chapter is written by Nada Savitch along with four people living with dementia who use technology in different ways: Tom Hawkins, Ann Johnson, Keith Oliver and Ken Clasper. Nada has drawn together some of the issues highlighted by the four authors as well as drawing on her own experience of supporting people with dementia to use and test different technologies.

Introduction

People with dementia are like other people – we all use technology in our everyday lives, sometimes without even noticing it. Technology means different things to different people. My co-authors have all defined it as things that help. But there can also be a resistance and even fear around the word 'technology'. There is also concern about technology replacing human contact. People with dementia and carers who contributed to the guide 'Getting equipped to tackle forgetfulness: Top tips for family and friends' (Foundation for Assistive Technology, Innovations in Dementia and Trent DSDC 2011) liked different terms, including 'equipment', 'gadgets' and 'devices'. Some people might include hearing aids as technology and others might include cars. But most people think of technology as electronic devices.

In this chapter, we discuss what everyday technology people use, some of the dementia-specific equipment people have come across, their feelings about using technology, the difficulties people have, some thoughts about design and support and some thoughts about the future.

Everyday technology

Some technology is very practical, some is vital for our wellbeing. In this respect, the way people with dementia use technology is the same as everyone else. Like most people's homes, the homes of the co-authors and most other people with dementia are full of technology. These include gadgets for entertainment such as TVs, radios and DVD players, but also household equipment such as washing machines, cookers and microwaves and, of course, the things that often spring to mind when you hear the word 'technology': computers, tablets and mobile phones.

What is obvious from the experiences of the co-authors and other people with dementia I have worked with is that everyone uses these technologies differently, and also that people's experiences are very different. Like the rest of the population, people with dementia have different needs for using technology. And for all of us, the design of technology can make it easy to use or frustrating.

Perhaps the main difference is that for people with dementia, those frustrations with design can be more pronounced and affect people's self-esteem more vividly. For example, not being able to use gadgets and equipment around the house changes people's roles in life and their relationships with family and friends. Another difference might be that people with dementia increasingly need more support and to receive this really need to be connected to other people. Technology can help people be connected and support interdependency. For example, using email or text messaging enables people to compose their thoughts before sending.

Another important point is that the significance of using everyday technology changes as the dementia progresses. The co-authors of this chapter are all still using everyday technologies in different ways, but what they are using and how they are using it has changed over time. People with dementia might also be more reliant on technology than other people to relieve boredom. Boredom is an issue for many people with dementia, especially when people find reading or following TV programmes difficult. Technology has the capacity to help alleviate boredom but also to increase feelings of isolation.

Dementia-specific technology

By definition, dementia is a progressive condition, and all the authors realise that and are, to a greater or lesser extent, planning for the future. Although they may not be using many products designed especially for people with dementia right now, they are aware of some of the products and are hopeful that technology will play a positive role in their lives in the future.

Technology that is more specialist in design often helps with memory, navigation and safety. But people with dementia are equally concerned about how equipment and gadgets could help with communication and entertainment. The authors are already using more everyday technology to help with reminders and the time of day, plus voice recorders. They also mention the increasing use of technology in health and social care, such as online consultations with a GP, tracking devices and sensors around the house.

Design of this equipment is key. Many engineers and designers (usually from outside the dementia field) tend to start by being very interested in what a particular technology can do, and then look for some way of trying it out, rather than starting with bottom-up research, which would show them what people want. The authors of this chapter also point out that many of the problems that they experience using technology are not to do with memory. Perceptual issues are also a real barrier to using many gadgets. The authors of this chapter point out that design is key for them to be able to use technology. It is easy, however, for researchers to lose touch with the beneficiaries of their work. In their guide 'Core Principles for Involving People with Dementia in Research', the Scottish Dementia Working Group (SDWG; 2013, p.8) say, 'We are often involved in answering research questions, but we are not often asked about research priorities.' The SDWG believe that research priorities shouldn't just be set by researchers, but they shouldn't just be set by people with dementia either. They think that people with dementia and researchers should work together in influencing knowledge about dementia.

Feelings about technology

All the authors are relatively positive about technology. They have used and continue to use technology and will try to use it and make the most of different equipment and gadgets. However, they all also talk about technology being a mixed blessing. In particular, people highlight being annoyed or being frustrated when they use technology. Sometimes this frustration is about the technology itself but often it is also that using technology highlights the changes in their abilities and needs because of dementia and its symptoms. However, there are also big positives. A major one for the authors is how technologies can help them to communicate and connect with others. In particular, many people with dementia find handwriting difficult. Typing can be easier than using a pen and paper, and voice recognition software can help. But in addition, technology can help people with spelling and grammar. It also allows people time to compose their thoughts and make sure they are represented by what has been typed.

The nature of dementia means that many people with dementia can feel lonely and bored. The authors of this chapter highlight how technology can keep people connected and entertained, but also that if they can't use the technology they may have to give up hobbies, interests, friends and activities. It is interesting that the authors are not worried about the ethics of using different technologies. But they are concerned that people with dementia should be more involved in design.

What makes 'technology' difficult

'It's a very bewildering world for everyone getting older... Nothing is simple anymore.' This is a quote from *Getting Equipped to Tackle Forgetfulness* (Foundation for Assistive Technology, Innovations in Dementia and Trent DSDC 2011, p.5). It reflects the views of the co-authors of this chapter, even if they are not very old. As dementia progresses, using some types of technology can become more difficult. The authors point out some design and accessibility issues, such as complexity and the use of passwords and codes, but also the difficulties that change – often a necessity in the technology world – presents to them. They also highlight some more hidden concerns around technology such as reliability, cost and exposure to fraud.

Complexity is probably the most obvious design concern for people with dementia. Some of the authors talk about giving up on complicated technology. Some people with dementia are able to ignore functionality that doesn't interest them, but this is not as easy as it sounds for most people. Lots of technology from computers to alarm systems rely on passwords or codes for security. Reliance on remembering passwords is an obvious issue for people with memory problems.

Many people with dementia report finding change of any sort difficult. Designing in a way that is similar to websites and other systems and devices can help (Savitch and Zaphiris 2007). But the authors also pointed out the confusion that goes with upgrades to operating systems (e.g. on a smartphone) and the unfamiliarity of everyday equipment that has changed beyond recognition, such as telephones.

A loss of confidence often accompanies a diagnosis of dementia, and people may feel more vulnerable. When a person with dementia puts trust in a piece of technology to support them, it is vitally important that the technology is reliable and does what it is supposed to do. For similar reasons, the cost of using technology is not a surprising concern; nor is concern about exposure to fraud and scams when using technology.

Support to use technology

There is no doubt that many people with dementia would continue to be active users of technology if they had more support (Stokes and Savitch 2011). However, the nature of that support is important. The authors of this chapter point out that support is not always available. People with dementia often do not have a family carer. Even where they do, there is no guarantee that the carer is confident using technology.

But support goes much further than having someone around. There is a lot of technology available and people need support to find out what technology might work for us as individuals (Savitch, Brooks and Wey 2012). It's important to know what is out there, to understand how much it would cost, maybe to try it before you buy or to read the reviews of others. But it is also important that installation and instructions are helpful, not more confusing.

Case study 7.1 Ken Clasper

Ken Clasper has a diagnosis of Lewy body dementia and also has hearing problems and chronic obstructive pulmonary disease (COPD). He is a well-known and well-read blogger about his experiences of living with long-term conditions (Clasper 2018). He and his wife Janice have been active in raising awareness of dementia for some years. Ken is an ambassador with the Lewy Body Society.

Ken's views on technology

Technology is a lovely thing, if you can use it and understand it these days.

I use technology most days, whether it's my mobile phone, tablet computer, or whether it's things like the voice-activated software on my computer, which is a great help on my bad days, when it's difficult to use a computer keyboard. This is a godsend, but it has its downside, because there are days when it fails to recognise my voice, so I have to spend time going over the course again teaching the equipment to understand what I am saying. This is often seen as part of Parkinson's disease, which is similar to Lewy body dementia. The tone of our voice changes on a regular basis.

Sometimes the problem is with reliability and sometimes with the unexpected. I was using a Fitbit but it upgraded itself without me knowing. I got very confused, and it was telling me stuff that wasn't right. Familiarity is good – but technology is always changing. I had to change mobile phone, and the font size was different which was really unhelpful. It's also disconcerting when a piece of technology talks to you. I'm happy with talking maps, but only when I'm expecting it. I wouldn't get on with one of those gadgets that talk to you all the time.

Another problem with mobile phones is the fear of overspending. I got a new deal with a new phone, which included extra data – but it was hidden so I was really concerned.

Children are growing up with various forms of technology these days, and perhaps they will adapt to newer forms of technology in the future, but I do wonder if they will be able to function without it when things go wrong.

When we go into supermarkets, we see modern technology at the checkouts, but if there is a power failure, the store has to close, because no one can add up without the technology any more. When I was young, the store staff added up your bill, usually on a piece of paper where it could be seen and checked, but those days have long gone. However, many elderly people have never come across some of this technology, and in some cases they may not want to use it. I confess that I don't cope with the self-service checkouts very well, and tend to join the big queues waiting to be served by real staff, rather than a machine.

There are so many possibilities for using technology to keep you occupied or active, but I do worry that soon it's going to get beyond the control of many elderly people, or those with a neurological illness.

I suppose the day will come when doctors' appointments could be done via Skype or telephone or even email, rather than face to face, and this will cause problems to those who don't cope with technology very well. These days we are told to order our prescriptions, and also arrange appointments over the Internet. I get confused doing this and my wife does not like it, so we do it the old way by going to the doctor's surgery.

However, many elderly people and those living with dementia, etc., are using technology at home to keep themselves active, in the hope of staving off the illness for a little bit longer.

But it worries me that technology is now being overused in many places, making it difficult for elderly people and those with neurological illnesses to keep up with constant changes.

Years ago, there were many complaints about the use of technology to track people with dementia, but in all honesty, everyone who uses a mobile phone is tracked by a satellite, so if you can use a mobile phone and be tracked, why is it so wrong to use it to track people with dementia? Because at the end of the day, it's for our safety, and is giving us the freedom to do whatever we want, without needing full-time carers with us. This gives us the freedom to do what we want, when we want, so we can live an active life without social workers or anyone else telling us what we can and can't do.

But technology is far reaching, and some people would be totally lost without it. I wouldn't be without my phone and tablet.

Technology needs to be manageable on a day-to-day basis, but it can be frustrating or annoying. What does annoy me, and I don't suppose I am alone, is the fact that companies keep changing their websites, and this in turn makes life so much harder for those of us whose brain is doing its own thing. It would be so much more helpful if gadgets were kept simple. I can use the microwave, but only on the basic settings. I've had to learn which ready meals are simple to cook. Although I use my tablet for blogging, I find cutting and pasting on the tablet difficult, so still use the large screen of the computer sometimes. I like to play games on the tablet to keep my brain active. In the same way, I like to use a camera with manual settings, although this is getting more difficult and frustrating now, so I sometimes use the camera on the phone.

Case study 7.2 Tom Hawkins

Tom has a diagnosis of vascular dementia. He was active in the local Lewisham Mind advocacy group and he and his wife Maureen are part of the ALWAYS group – an advisory group of people with dementia and carers for the IDEAL research project at the University of Exeter.

Tom and Maureen's view of technology

Technology is getting more and more difficult to use. Tom used to be the more tech-minded of us, so it's getting more confusing.

We think of technology in the broadest sense. It should mean anything that helps us, but some of the technology we use is too complicated and unfamiliar. When Tom was first diagnosed we got a tablet computer, but it was too difficult for both of us.

Everyday technology is still OK for us. Modern kitchen gadgets are helpful – the toast pops up and the kettle turns itself off. But some technology is too technical and too confusing.

Tom's hearing aids are great when it's calm and he can hear the birds. But he often takes them out when thing get too loud – like when children are around.

We like things that are familiar. Tom prefers to use the old-fashioned house telephone that looks like a phone. When the phone rings he'll pick that one up, but not our new cordless phone. It's too complicated, you have to use the buttons and it doesn't look like a phone. But the new phone is great because it blocks any number that's not in the address book.

Some gadgets we have are too similar. We share the chores around the house and garden – but sometimes Tom gets the vacuum cleaner and the lawn mower mixed up. They look so similar and do similar things – inside and out!

We do sometimes hear about technology that might help. It might be useful to do shopping online. We've also heard about tracking devices, which Tom would like to use to enable him to go out without me worrying – but I'm not confident enough to use the computer to set it up.

Codes are getting more difficult. Tom can still set the burglar alarm, but bank cards are trickier.

Although Tom is using less technology, he doesn't feel like he's missing out: 'Don't see the need for it – the generation now want everything!'

The future might see technological developments that could help – but it's difficult to know. Tom doesn't want a robot carer – he says it might 'clunk'. Not being able to drive is really difficult for Tom, but we're not sure driverless cars would help. The issue is more about not being able to do things you used to, rather than getting from A to B. It's difficult for us to get used to new technology. The neighbours have a robotic hoover, but we wouldn't trust it to get into the corners!

Case study 7.3 Ann Johnson

Ann Johnson travels around the country giving talks to raise awareness of dementia.

Ann moved into a care home in Greater Manchester soon after she was diagnosed with dementia at the age of 52. She is a retired nurse tutor and since her diagnosis, she has received an MBE for her services to healthcare. She has co-edited a book on social research methods in dementia studies (Keady *et al.* 2018).

Ann's views of technology

Technology is all about helping people to function. The simple things in life make things easier for us. I use technology to help me to keep connected and able to give my talks. The technology that means the most to me is my mobile phone, my voice recorder and email.

I use my voice recorder at night to leave myself reminders about what to do the next day. Before I go to bed I just press the record button and speak into it. I play it every morning. It's fun to see what's on it! It might be details of a meeting or someone visiting, or what time to get the bus in the morning. It's usually a list of things to do for the day. I've had it a long time, it's just a simple thing I bought from Argos. I can't really remember why I bought it – it just seemed like a good idea. Someone suggested it to me, as I was worried about forgetting things. It's very simple – one button to record and one to play. When the original one stopped working, I got another one.

I used to record all the talks which I gave, but I don't any more be-cause I lost them all when the machine broke. That's annoying because I don't remember what I say to people. I'm happy with what I say at the time, but I don't remember it. I write my talks down now.

My phone and computer are only useful for me to keep in touch with people. I'd be lost without my phone and email. Without them, I'd lose contact with people and that would not be good. My mobile phone is as simple as it can be. It's not a smartphone because I only use it to make and receive phone calls and for text messages. I can't do handwriting any more, so prefer to type. It takes me a long time to write a text because I don't like getting words wrong and won't send the message until I'm happy. In the same way, I only use the computer to send email. I can handle email, but not much else on the computer.

Some aspects of technology do worry me. I can use email and my phone because it's all set up for me the way I like it. I couldn't cope with a smartphone. I get a lot of rubbish emails. I know enough not to click on any link I don't know. The cost of technology could also be a concern – I've got a fixed contract for my broadband and phone.

Living in a care home means that I am aware of some of the technology that might help me in the future. I know I'm getting worse and one day I won't know where I am. I'd be happy to use sensors and tracking technology if they helped me. I know there is a place for that sort of technology if it keeps you safe. I think cameras might have a place to make sure you are getting the care you need and not being mistreated, but we don't have that problem here.

I have a talking clock – but it's a bit confusing. The clock face is set to the 24-hour clock, but when it speaks it uses the 12-hour clock. I have to press a button to get it to speak, so I don't use it very often. But I do find reading a clock face difficult which gets me down and frustrated. It's not good to see myself disappearing.

Technology does need to be reliable. I used to carry information with me through a company called ContactMe. It felt like a safety net for me when I went out. But now the company has folded, so I'll have to rely on the tongue in my head if I get lost.

I also use technology for leisure. I find reading difficult, so I watch TV and listen to the radio in the morning in bed and also use audio books on CD which I play through the TV. The radio has one button and comes on to the station I like, and I know which buttons I use on the TV remote and ignore all the rest. Bad design is frustrating and annoying – I have an alarm clock that you have to turn around to turn it off.

The simplest things are the most useful. And good support is vital. I rely on the man who delivers my printer cartridge to change it for me. He's very patient with me.

In truth the word 'technology' worried me. I can't understand a lot of it. If you can explain it to me, that's fine, but if I don't understand it, I'll question it.

Case study 7.4 Keith Oliver

Keith Oliver was diagnosed with Alzheimer's disease in 2010. He is an ambassador for the Alzheimer's Society and is involved in their research network. He is the Dementia Service-User Envoy for Kent and Medway NHS and Social Care Partnership Trust. Keith works tirelessly with different organisations and projects to raise awareness about dementia. His book *Walk the Walk, Talk the Talk* was published in 2016 and *Dear Alzheimer's* was published by Jessica Kingsley Publishers in 2019.

Keith's views on technology

I see positive and negatives in my use of technology. Sometimes I think that technology can be liberating and a positive experience if it helps you to do the things you want to do. However, on the other hand it can cause frustration and reinforce feelings of inability. Realising that you need assistive technology to function might have a negative impact on confidence and self-esteem. And forgetting how things work or forgetting to use something can be frustrating and upsetting.

It is important that technology is viewed as an aid and a tool to support us – but not to take over, and certainly not as a replacement for human intervention. When I was first diagnosed I wouldn't answer the telephone, but I now think that was less to do with the technology and more because I was worried about the conversation or not remembering the conversation.

I am certainly put off using technology that I find difficult. For example, my enthusiasm for listening to music has diminished as the dementia progresses, at least in part because I have difficulty using the CD player. There is often an expectation that support is always available – from family, carers or friends. This is not always the case – and sometimes family and friends might know less about the technology in question than I do.

My use of technology is changing because of the dementia. I find change difficult. We recently got a new TV and I don't understand the remote control. It has too many buttons that are not needed, it's very confusing. It's particularly confusing, because with this new TV the volume levels are not displayed on the TV screen. It's not something I thought to check before I bought it. Technology is constantly changing and so we need to think about its place in dementia care. For example, people might want to put an electric kettle on the hob – when they might be perfectly OK with an old-fashioned whistling kettle. I use a computer regularly, but I'm always concerned about upgrades. I can't remember my mobile phone number even after nine years.

I want to help around the house and still use the tumble dryer and the hoover, but I no longer do any clothes washing or cooking – and that's entirely due to the technology involved. I used to cook quite a lot, but my confidence has gone completely and I'm fearful because I'm easily distracted. The Fire Service gave us timers, but I can't remember how to use them. I would really struggle to eat properly if I didn't live with my wife.

But, on the other hand, I would be lost without my computer and my mobile phone as these are vital for my work as an activist in the dementia field. I find technology such as computers and mobile phones vital for connecting to others, contributing to society and getting stuff done. It's part of my routine and I've grown up with it, but it's rapidly changing. At times it's frustrating to think that I used to teach with technology – I wasn't a 'geek' but I was responsible for implementing whiteboard technology.

I still feel that technology is a means to an end. I find communication technologies such as email and text messages can be both useful and alienating. Written communication can be challenging for me – I don't write as quickly or as well as I want to. My handwriting has deteriorated and I find spelling increasingly difficult. It is easier to correct text on a screen. But it can be painful for me to write an email as I want to get it right and it can be very demoralising when it isn't right. I want to keep hold of the 'professional' Keith Oliver. I also find it frustrating when professionals who I work with insist on using technology that I am finding difficult. I'm involved in different projects where lots of different professionals communicate by email. I find it very difficult to follow conversations and trails conducted via email. If I could I would use text messages as it's easier to keep track and manage communication.

When designing or using technology it is important to include the experience of the person with dementia. People with dementia need to be involved in the development stage of design and testing prototypes, not just to endorse a product that already exists.

People often forget how many people with dementia, including me, have problems with spatial awareness. I've wrecked computers by hitting the keyboard too hard or by knocking water over it. I also have problems using the microwave because I see the dials differently, depending on which angle I'm looking at it.

Another thing I find difficult is passwords and codes. I first realised that something was wrong with me when I couldn't remember the code for the alarm system at the school where I was head teacher. Sometimes I find remembering words easier than number codes. I could keep a book of passwords, but I'd probably forget where I've put it.

Technology needs to be reliable. A long time ago, I trialled a tracking device as part of a university project. If I got lost, I was to contact the call centre and they would be able to tell me where I was. Sometimes it worked exactly, but one time it placed me three-quarters of a mile from where I really was. That experience really knocked my confidence.

Although I don't use technology that uses sensors around the house, it's reassuring to know that the technology is out there and could help in the future when I might need it.

Having said that, I feel that there is sometimes too much emphasis on technology when research projects are funded. Technology should be a part of research, but not the sole element. It might be naïve to think that big technology companies have a social conscience, but some are more socially aware than others. Maybe mainstream technology will not be dementia friendly until we start using our financial power. In many ways people with dementia are reliant on being a 'fashionable' cause.

It's important to encourage people who sell technology to understand the needs of people with dementia so that they can support them. We need support to make good decisions when purchasing everyday technology, but there is also a role for retailers to show people how technology works (as part of the delivery process) as well as how to use the technology to its best. I know that people like me will forget how to use kit, so good instructions are important and good tech support. User manuals are now either online or in many different languages – we need step-by-step instructions, preferably with pictures. In particular, I often need help just to turn something on.

Technology is becoming more prevalent in everyday life. Automated telephone exchanges where you have to press different keys for different options make it almost impossible to contact many organisations. I don't use the Internet for banking or shopping – this is partly a confidence issue and partly because of a fear of fraud.

Technology is also often finding its way into health and social care. Technologies such as telehealth and telecare have a place, but they need to enhance not replace human support. It's particularly important for health professionals such as occupational therapists (OTs) to understand different technologies and be able to support people with dementia to use it.

The future

The authors of this chapter are optimistic about the future. They hope that technology will be available that will support them and others like them. It seems nowadays that every new technology from telehealth to robots and driverless cars is associated with supporting people with dementia. However, design which does not involve potential users risks delivering products or services that people cannot understand, with the result that they do not use it, or which fails to accommodate any deterioration in their condition, which means it is abandoned. Therefore, product design needs to be flexible and robust enough to address changing needs.

A lot of design for people with dementia focuses on a deficit approach, that is, designing products for what people can't do. Good designs work with what people can do and seeks to support them. Many products that are designed for people with dementia focus on keeping people safe. Although this is important, more design is needed around encouraging greater independence, supporting leisure activities and helping people to have fun.

Putting the needs and aspirations of people with dementia at the heart of the design process is fundamental. Finding out what people with dementia want to do with products or technology is hard. But it's worth the effort to find out what people with dementia want from products, what they know about what's available and how they use the products or technology that they do have. Designers really need to focus on finding out from people with dementia what's important in their lives and what they are finding difficult to continue to do in their lives, and then looking at how technology can address these challenges.

Take-home points

* People with dementia use and rely on technology.

* Different people use technology differently.

* Using technology can be frustrating, especially as dementia progresses.

* Involving people with dementia in the design of technology is vital.

* Support is important, but more nuanced than just relying on family carers.

Acknowledgements

We would like to thank all the people with dementia and projects we have been involved with, for example the ALWAYS group at the IDEAL project, and the people who support us every day. Particular thanks go to Christine Redfearn, Maureen Hawkins, Rosemary Oliver and Janice Clasper.

PART 3

Technology Ecosystem for Dementia

Chapter 8

Technology for Families of People with Dementia

Dr Emma Wolverson, *Clinical Psychologist and Clinical Lecturer,*
School of Health and Social Work, Faculty of Health Sciences, University of Hull, UK

Rosie Dunn, *Research Assistant, School of Health and Social Work,*
Faculty of Health Sciences, University of Hull, UK

Caroline White, *Research Associate, School of Health and*
Social Work, Faculty of Health Sciences, University of Hull, UK

Introduction

Caring for another human being is an endeavour requiring incredible skill, dedication and patience. Family carers[1] juggle many roles: counsellor, secretary, home help, cheerleader – the list goes on! So much of what carers do is intuitive; anticipating a person's needs and always walking that delicate tightrope between knowing when to step in and help, and when to sit back and encourage independence.

It might seem odd, then, to think of technology assisting in such a complicated and skilful task. Indeed, technology is certainly not the be-all and end-all of caring; there could never be a robot skilful enough to meet a person's needs in the unassuming and personal way that you do. What technology can offer, though, is assistance and support – if you find the right thing for you. This is the key, as the last thing you want to do is add to your stress levels!

---

1   Caring for and supporting people with dementia is a role that is undertaken by many people, such as family members, friends and neighbours, some of whom do not think of themselves as carers at all. In this chapter we refer to 'family carers' and 'relatives', but recognise that other people provide care and support too.

Technology for family carers is a massive growth industry. It is seen as being a solution flexible enough to meet the needs of the modern family, capable of supporting the growing numbers of carers juggling paid work and family life with caring, sometimes from a distance. What is available is constantly changing and more technology is being researched and tested all the time. As such, what we present here is as true as it can be today, but you should bear in mind that next week there will probably be something new on the market! Additionally, as the needs of the person that you care for change over time, you might want to revisit this chapter and take another look at what's available.

With that in mind, this chapter is designed to give you a brief overview and introduction, hopefully opening your eyes to some areas where technology might help you. Our aim is simply to get you thinking, and so while we will provide some examples, they are by no means exhaustive – you should go away and find out more about anything that catches your interest. We include products here as examples so you can research further; we are not providing any recommendations or endorsing specific products. We have included both high-tech and low-tech options because we have found that carers often don't have the time to search the Internet and find out what technologies are available and so often make use of what they are familiar with – often to very good effect!

Working out what might be useful to you

With so much technology out there, how can you work out what might be helpful for you? Recommendations from friends or family can be helpful, but what works for someone else might not work for you. The best place to start is to think about what the main challenges are that you need more help with – what is it you want the technology to do for you? Do you need to be alerted when the person you support leaves the house? Do you need a system that reminds the person where you are when you have popped out to the shops or into the garden?

Here are some other important things to consider when thinking about what you might choose:

- *Whether you live with the person or not.* Some technologies are designed to be used remotely; others need you to be there to turn them on/off.

- *Where the person is in their dementia journey.* Some technology is great for helping you to support people in the early stages of dementia, but for a person with more advanced difficulties the technology could be confusing or too difficult – for instance, alarms and voice reminders might frighten some people. Dementia is of course a progressive illness, so over time a piece of technology might stop being useful, or you might face new challenges that you need to find solutions for.

- *Sensory needs.* Think about your sensory needs and abilities and those of the person with dementia – eyesight and hearing problems might mean some technologies are problematic. There are lots of technologies specifically designed for those with hearing and visual impairments that can be helpful – for example, pill boxes, doorbells that flash and talking books.

- *Cost.* The cost of different technologies and gadgets varies significantly. Some can be purchased for a one-off payment – some apps, for example, cost only a few pounds, whereas some systems cost hundreds. Other equipment requires a monthly subscription fee. You need to think about whether the technology could save you money in the long run; perhaps if it reduces the need for a care package at home. Is it worth the investment if it helps keep the person you care for independent and improves your mood and wellbeing?

- *How comfortable are you with technology?* Think about how easy the technology will be to install and maintain, and who you can get support from to set it up (family, friends, the company providing it). What support is there if the technology stops working?

- *Do you need any infrastructure for the technology to work?* For instance, does it require a telephone landline or Internet access? If so, is your Internet fast enough? Will the company need to come and install anything? If they do, how will the person living with dementia feel about this?

- *Time.* While technology can often save you time and effort in the long run, you have to be prepared to invest some time when you are first putting it in place. You may need time to train the person to get used to the technology and for a while you may need to remind them to use it until it becomes part of their routine.

How do you find out what's available?

A simple start can be to do an Internet search – there is lots of information out there, some of it reliable and some not. There are some good online resources and we have listed some places to look at the end of this chapter. Some larger companies have YouTube channels where they use videos to demonstrate technology and what it can do.

Talk to other carers and professionals and ask them what they have heard of, what they use and what they recommend. Some memory clinics, memory cafés and assistive technology and social care centres will have technology available to show you, which you may be able to borrow to see if it can work for you at home. Occupational therapists (OTs) can be of great support in thinking about what technology might be right for you. OTs can be accessed via health providers and social care services. There are also community-based resources, such as local libraries, that help people to learn to use the Internet, computers or touchscreen devices, if you think your own skills or familiarity with technology might be a barrier.

Now we will move on to share an overview of the main areas where technology has been developed for family members who support a relative with dementia. We have divided these into sections on using technology to:

- find information online

- look after yourself as a carer

- make everyday life easier

- provide reassurance and peace of mind

- enjoy time with the person you care for.

We then share some findings from our own research project developing a website for people living with dementia and carers; this highlighted the importance of privacy and ethics, which for some family carers has been a barrier to using technology.

Finding information online

Family carers have many information needs. However, they may struggle to find information, and require information that is accessible to them and meets their needs in a timely way (Allen, Cain and Meyer 2018; Carer's Trust 2015). Furthermore, they may not be aware of all the information that could be useful to them. These difficulties were summed up by a family carer in our research (see below) who stated:

> In the beginning when you're faced with a diagnosis…where do you go to get help? What are the questions that you have to ask? Because you are on your own with this, nobody tells you, 'Oh, you need to contact this person, you need to ask that question' – you don't know what question. So basically, me and Google became very good friends. (Daughter of a person living with dementia)

The Internet is a useful source of information, which includes factual information, and online forums and blogs, in which carers share information and advice. However, the quality and reliability of online information is variable. Therefore, there are a number of questions to consider when seeking information online (National Center for Complementary and Integrative Health 2018; NHS Choices 2015):

- Who produced the information? Information from well-established, well-known organisations and statutory healthcare providers, as well as government websites, can usually be expected to be reliable and accurate.

- When was the information produced or updated? Some information (especially information about medical interventions, welfare benefits, legislation, local organisations and resources) may become out of date and so unreliable. Therefore, it is important to check when the information was produced. Similarly, some information is country-, state- or local council-specific, so it is also useful to check the area covered.

- Is the information consistent across more than one website? This may suggest that the information is more likely to be reliable.

When seeking information online, it is important to be aware that it will not all apply to your personal situation. There are many different types of dementia, and huge differences in how individuals are affected. Experiences shared on blogs and online forums are often very personal reflections. Reading the experiences of people 'in the same boat' can provide helpful insights and advice; however, it is important to consider any information and advice in the context of your own circumstances, needs and values, as well as the situation of the person you support.

While there is much valuable information online, should you become upset, concerned or confused as a result of information searches, it is important to contact a professional or organisation with expertise in dementia or carers' issues, for clarification and reassurance.

The Internet can also provide information in the form of online training, enabling carers to develop knowledge and confidence (Hattink *et al.* 2015; Marziali and Garcia 2011). Such training may include providing information about dementia or specific medical and care needs. Online training can enable carers to access information and learning from their own homes, at the times most convenient to them — especially helpful for carers who are working or cannot leave the person they support (Hattink *et al.* 2015; Marziali and Donahue 2006). In addition to providing training materials, some online training resources also enable carers to share experiences and knowledge with other carers through online chat or video links, enabling carers to gain both information and emotional support (Marziali and Donahue 2006; Marziali and Garcia 2011).

Looking after yourself

All too often carers end up pushing their own needs to one side as they struggle to make time for themselves (Lorenz *et al.* 2017). Yet it is so important to look after yourself and to stay fit and well in order to keep providing care and support. The UK Alzheimer's Society (2016b) have a brilliant fact sheet about looking after yourself. You may also want to consider how technology can help you find some time for yourself and look after your own wellbeing.

Managing tasks and prioritising

Using the Internet to help with online banking to pay bills, or shopping online, can save a lot of time and effort. There are also lots of apps available to help you manage your time and prioritise; 'to do' list apps are very popular and can send you reminders and even rewards for completing tasks! You can also set reminders and alerts in your calendar on your smartphone. The great thing about electronic lists and reminders is that they can be shared with others, which can be a useful way of getting other people to help out.

Talking to others

Talking about your feelings and experiences with others can be really beneficial (Alzheimer's Society 2014). Talking with other carers can be extremely helpful as you can share advice and ideas with others who might understand what you are going through. Online carers' support groups or discussion forums, such as the Alzheimer's Society's Talking Point, can be a valuable source of support, especially for those who can't get out to groups or memory cafés (Newbronner *et al.* 2013).

Involve others and ask for help

Don't be afraid to ask for help and support when you need it. Sometimes people don't offer to help because they don't know what they can do or because they think you are managing well. There are apps to help you share and coordinate care with others. These let others see what tasks and appointments are coming up and put their name by them. You can share notes with each other about your thoughts regarding the person's health and wellbeing – so you can all track things like their medication or pain levels together. They give you a way to collect and share summaries of medical appointments so you don't have to phone round everyone after each appointment. An example of an app like this is 'Jointly', which was developed by Carers UK. Even something as simple as a shared shopping list can let other people know what they need to pick up before they visit. Similarly, technology can provide a means to coordinate care between professional healthcare services like home carers. Such systems are likely to increase in the future as health services become 'paperless' and routinely use online health records. Ask home care providers if they use any shared care apps.

Think positively

Sometimes it can be hard to see the positive things that you are achieving in your caring role. Writing things down (even small things) can be useful. Then when you are having a bad day, these can remind you that there will be better times. Online journals are really popular; you can choose to keep your journal private or to share your experiences with others. Gratitude journals have been demonstrated to increase wellbeing (Emmons and Mishra 2011); these are available online and send you a daily reminder to think about one thing you are grateful for.

Take a break

There is growing evidence of the value of relaxation and mindfulness-based approaches in helping to improve family carers' wellbeing (e.g. Whitebird *et al.* 2013). Finding time to stop and reflect can be hard, but there are lots of relaxation, meditation and deep breathing apps that you can use at home – Headspace,[2] for example, is a very popular app.

Sleep

Sleep is important as it helps the brain and body recover. It can be difficult if the person you care for has disturbed nights or if you find it hard to switch off. Apps have been designed to help improve sleep by looking at your sleep cycle, and helping you relax and drift off.

If you think you need more help and support, the first person to contact is your GP, and most now offer online services to their patients enabling you to book appointments and order repeat prescriptions online, making it easier to interact with your GP and access services.

---

2   www.headspace.com

Making everyday life easier

Sometimes people living with dementia lose confidence in their memory ability and begin to rely on their carers to become their memory. It can often feel easier for carers to take over tasks and household activities, especially if feeling under pressure or time-limited. However, as carers it is important to empower the person living with dementia to have confidence to continue doing things for themselves and promote their independence for as long as possible.

There is a range of technology and gadgets available to help make day-to-day life easier and reduce feelings of stress for carers. Many people have developed systems that work for them, such as using wall calendars or diaries. Therefore, it is important that any additional technology fits in with your everyday life and routine, as well as meeting your particular needs. There are some great, low-cost gadgets available that carers have found helpful when supporting people living with dementia, as well as in reducing the everyday stresses and strains that life brings. You can find more information about technologies that help around the home in Chapter 4, 'Life at Home and Technology with Dementia'.

Managing medication

One example of how technology might help to make everyday life easier is in managing medication. Taking medications can be difficult and a source of worry if not managed correctly, as it can lead to further health problems. You might have your own medication to manage too, so it's important that systems are in place to get it right.

Simple pill boxes (also known as 'nomads' or 'dosette boxes') are widely available to help people organise and remember their medication and to provide reassurance to those worried about forgetting. Automatic pill dispensers are devices that alert users to take their medication and open automatically at the right day or time. At other times the box is locked, reducing the chance of accidentally taking too many pills. An alarm often continues to sound until the person has taken their tablets and closed the compartment.

It is advisable for people to seek advice from a local pharmacy to find out which type of box would best suit their needs, as well as to see if they offer a service to pre-fill the boxes. This can help ease the pressure on families and reduces the chance of taking the wrong medication, especially for those who take lots of different tablets. However, being reminded still doesn't guarantee that people will actually take them. It might be that people get side-tracked or that they can't get used to a new device buzzing. Some automatic pill dispensers have tried to tackle this problem by sending a notification to carers when the person hasn't taken their medication.

Reassurance and peace of mind

One of the biggest concerns for carers is the safety of the person they support. This might be a particular worry when carers are not with the person, for example if they live somewhere else or when they are away from home. Table 8.1 includes some information about technologies that can help people living with dementia to manage tasks more safely, providing reassurance to carers.

Table 8.1 Technology that may offer reassurance and peace of mind to people living with dementia and their carers

Technology that helps the user	
Name of technology	*How it can help*
Detectors	Makes people aware of dangers, such as fire, carbon monoxide, flooding, risk of scalding
Pillow alerts	Vibrates if there is a dangerous situation such as a fire; especially helpful if the person is deaf or hard of hearing
Automatic shut-off devices	Turns off cookers (if gas is accidentally left on), or taps which have been left running
Plug sensors	Can help reduce risk of flooding or scalding by monitoring water temperature
Video door entry systems	Allows people to see who is at the door before answering
Motion sensors	Detects where a person is situated in the home, and uses pre-recorded messages to remind people to lock the front door or turn off the oven

Bogus caller button	Enables the person to call for help if a stranger tries to access their home
Lifeline	Alerts others if the person falls or needs help (the user presses a button on a pendant or wristwatch)
Bed/chair occupancy sensors	Alerts others if the person does not return (to their bed or chair) in a given period of time
Motion sensors	Monitors a person's movements in the home, such as number of times a person gets up in the night or leaves a door open ('Just Checking' is a UK example of a monitoring system used in a person's home)
Tracking devices, e.g. GPS devices and apps	These enable carers to track where the person is, enabling people to go out and about, while reducing carer anxiety. Some apps have 'geofencing' that alerts others if the person goes beyond a set perimeter

Some technologies monitor people quite closely. While this can reduce worries for carers, it is important to consider and talk about how the person living with dementia feels about this. It is important to look for a solution that feels comfortable for the carer and the person with dementia.

Monitoring your relative's care

Some carers experience anxiety and concern about their relative's wellbeing and safety when they are receiving support from paid carers (for example in a care home or from a home care service). While it is important to remember that much care is of high quality, some services have been found to offer poor standards of care. There have been a number of high-profile cases where families have used surveillance technologies to monitor their relative's care and support, and have uncovered poor or abusive practices. The Care Quality Commission (CQC; regulator of health and social care services in England) has drawn up advice for carers who are considering using surveillance technologies, such as video cameras, audio recording equipment or motion sensors (Care Quality Commission 2015). Before exploring surveillance technologies, they note the importance of sharing any concerns about the service with the care provider (or an outside agency); they may take steps to address your concerns, meaning that you may not need to undertake your own monitoring and surveillance.

If you are considering using surveillance technologies you should think about how these impact on the privacy of other people, including your relative, any other residents, staff and visitors to the home. You should seek the agreement of your relative; if they do not have the capacity to provide this, you should consider whether this is likely to be in their best interests. This includes, for example, considering their personality, past views and wishes, current views and feelings, and the views of others who know them well (Alzheimer's Society 2015). If your relative lives in a care or nursing home, you should ensure you minimise the impact on other people by only using surveillance technologies in your relative's room, and avoiding communal areas.

The CQC also advise that you check whether your relative's care home has a policy on using recording equipment. It is also important to be aware of the possibility that others may consider legal action if they have been recorded, using human rights or data protection legislation. You may wish to seek legal advice prior to setting up surveillance equipment, to consider any potential legal risks. You also need to store the information recorded securely and only share this with others who have a legitimate reason to view this.

In the event that you uncover poor or abusive practices, you need to share these with practitioners and agencies that can support you and take steps to ensure the safety of your relative (and others). This might include service regulators, social workers, a local authority Adult Safeguarding Team (in the UK) or the police if you believe a crime has been committed. Charitable organisations (such as Action on Elder Abuse in the UK[3]) may also be able to provide valuable advice and support.

Managing finances

Ensuring that individuals' money is managed safely is a role frequently undertaken by carers. Online banking could help to monitor and track bills and payments. Carers could set up standing orders or direct debits for someone living with dementia, so that they do not have to worry about remembering to pay bills. Pre-paid debit cards mean that people

3   www.elderabuse.org.uk

can still go out and pay for things, but there is a limit set on how much they can spend. This can help people to still feel independent and in control of their finances but reduces the chance of overspending. If you are considering taking steps to help with managing your relative's finances, you may need to consider your legal position; this may include, for example, making arrangements to hold a Power of Attorney (in the UK) to authorise you to make decisions about and manage finances (Alzheimer's Society 2016a).

Sometimes, people with dementia can be targeted and at risk of fraudulent scams. There are some steps you can use to reduce these risks, for example you can block nuisance telephone calls or set up call screening, preventing people from being misled with cold calls or scams.

Spending time together and keeping in touch

People are sometimes concerned that technologies may replace human contact and interaction. However, technologies can also enable people with dementia and carers to connect with each other and enjoy time together.

Remembering together

People with dementia are often better able to remember past rather than recent events (Alzheimer's Society 2016c). Remembering past times can be an enjoyable way of spending time together, providing opportunities for communication and interaction. The Internet can be a rich source of material to help elicit memories and stories from an individual's past (Learner 2013). Websites can enable pictures, video footage, maps, music, and TV and film clips to be easily and quickly retrieved, such as the BBC RemArc site. Online photos may provide useful substitutes if the person with dementia has lost (or never had) photos of significant times and places (Critten and Kucirkova 2017). Some museums and businesses have online archives with useful pictures and information which may prompt memories and discussion.

Digital technologies can enable the creation and storage of material about a person's past. For example, touchscreen technologies such as tablets allow users to download material online, take photos, create captions and make audio recordings (for example of the person speaking about their memories; Critten and Kucirkova 2017). Apps can help organise material and enable the creation of online life story books (Critten and Kucirkova 2017). This can be an enjoyable activity, enabling families to see beyond the person's dementia, and can create a resource which can be shared with other family members, as well as any future carers (Critten and Kucirkova 2017; Kellett *et al.* 2010).

Music can also be a powerful trigger for memories, with music and songs often linked to memories of special occasions (Evans, Garabedien and Bray 2017; Playlist for Life n.d.). Listening to favourite music together can be an enjoyable activity for people living with dementia and carers, promoting interaction and reminiscence (Evans *et al.* 2017). The UK charity Playlist for Life provides valuable information about creating a playlist of significant music for people living with dementia. They suggest identifying music associated with important past times such as childhood, weddings, family parties and holidays, as well as TV theme tunes, which may elicit memories for the person. The Internet (for example sites such as YouTube) can help locate music which can be played or stored on a laptop, iPad or MP3 player.

It is important to remember that while reminiscing can help people share happy memories, it can sometimes evoke painful memories, which the person may not wish to discuss; any feelings of sadness should be acknowledged, but the person should not be pressed to pursue such memories (Thompson 2017).

Online resources for enjoying leisure time

There are a range of online games and activities which can allow people with dementia and carers to enjoy spending time together. These include online jigsaws, games such as patience, and puzzles such as word searches, crosswords and Sudoku, as well as 'brain training games'. These can enable people to try out new activities and challenges, as well as enjoy existing activities in new ways. Some of these resources are discussed in greater depth in Chapter 6, 'Leisure Activities and Technology with Dementia'.

Keeping in touch

Technologies can help families and people with dementia who do not live together keep in touch when apart. Communicating using the telephone can become a problem for many people. However, there are simple adaptations that can help you and your relative keep in touch by phone. Adapted telephones display large numbers or pictures and allow you to store frequently used telephone numbers – these are saved under a picture or photo related to the person, making it easy for people to call others with one touch of a button.

Video phones or the Internet (using facilities such as Skype or FaceTime) may facilitate communication and contact between carers and people living with dementia, and enhance interaction, in comparison with conventional telephones. Research on the use of video phones (Savenstedt, Brulin and Sandman 2003) found that the ability to see the person with dementia helped carers see how their relative was feeling, which provided reassurance, as well as enabling them to see that the person was listening and engaged. Similarly, the ability to see loved ones via video chat may help people living with dementia feel connected to their families and friends (Tinder Foundation 2016). People with dementia may require support to manage video chat (Savenstedt *et al.* 2003), so it may be useful to consider whether there is someone close by who can help them use the technology. For online video chat it is important to check that the person has an Internet connection (Social Care Institute for Excellence 2017), especially for people living in care homes, as not all provide Wi-Fi access for residents (Learner 2013).

Some people with dementia can develop speech problems, making it difficult for them to communicate. An application called 'Talking Mats' allows users to select a picture to let others know how they feel or if there is something they want or need. This can reduce feelings of frustration and isolation, and also improve relationships with family, friends and carers.

Case study 8.1 CaregiversPro-MMD: The importance of privacy and security when sharing information online

CaregiversPro-MMD is a social networking and information website currently being developed in partnership with people with memory problems and carers living in Europe (see Figure 8.1). The purpose of the website is to enable people to find useful information, as well as reducing isolation through participating in an online community, in which people can talk to other carers or people experiencing memory problems.

Research has found that services post-diagnosis are often 'patchy', so carers and people with dementia may lack support and information (Mountain and Craig 2012); it is hoped that CaregiversPro-MMD can help to address this gap and meet the needs of both carers and people living with dementia.

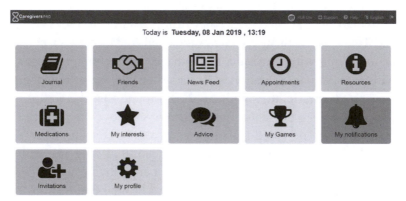

Figure 8.1 A screenshot of the CaregiversPro-MMD home screen

At the point of writing, the research is ongoing and people have been using the website to make connections, find out information and enjoy online leisure activities. One carer commented that they have gained 'friends at the touch of a button and help of all kinds – life is worth living after all'.

The development of the website has included ongoing discussions with people living with dementia and carers to inform the design, development and content of the website. From these discussions, one of the barriers identified to people taking up technology solutions was that some people were nervous about sharing information online, and were unclear about how to keep their information private online and reduce risks of information being misused. They also recognised that sharing information with others in a similar situation could be helpful, but also might cause worry or stress for some.

From the information shared by families we have identified a number of useful points for carers to consider if they or their relatives are joining online forums or searching for information online. These include the following:

- Think about what information you are happy to share online, and what information you prefer to keep private. For example, you may not feel comfortable and secure sharing information about medical matters or finances.

- Some sites have privacy settings so that you can choose who reads information you post. It is useful to familiarise yourself with the privacy settings, and choose the ones which are right for you.

- Some people living with dementia who took part in the research were not familiar with the idea of privacy when online. It may be useful to discuss with your relative what information they want to share, think together about any potential risks and see if they need help to set up privacy settings.

- Although lots of useful information can be shared online, sometimes people can be offensive or unkind. Some sites have a moderator who checks that people are not posting inappropriate information or comments. It may be useful to check whether a site is moderated or enables you to report inappropriate material.

- You and the person you support may have different interests and be at different stages in terms of the information and advice you want. Depending on your readiness to consider information about living with dementia you may want to do this together, or you may find that this is something you need to do alone, at least initially.

- It may also be helpful to look at online forums or social networking sites before joining to see if you feel comfortable with the information and the way it is presented.

Overall it is important to think about what information to share online, and how you share that information, to protect privacy and dignity both for you and the person you care for. One carer shared some really useful advice:

With respect for my mum I wouldn't discuss her real personal stuff. The general stuff, the ideas, 'I've bought this' or 'I got this piece of equipment' or whatever, I mean I might talk about me, 'I've had a hard day today,' or something like that, but nothing that's confidential.

Balancing the needs of carers and people with dementia

Some of the technologies we have described might benefit both carers and people living with dementia; others (such as apps to enable care to be coordinated) may mainly benefit carers while having little direct impact on people with dementia. However, our research suggests that there is potential for carers and people living with dementia to view technologies in very different ways. For example, carers have reported that tracking devices help provide peace of mind when the person they support is out and about. In contrast, some people with dementia have reported reservations about such technologies, not liking the feeling that they are being watched and sometimes finding the devices alarming or confusing, or even feeling less safe when they are using them (Robinson *et al.* 2007). Therefore, there are a number of issues to consider (Clark and McGee-Lennon 2011; Godwin 2012):

- How does the person living with dementia feel about the proposed technology? What, if any, concerns do they have? For example, are they worried that if monitors are installed they are being watched, or that other people will visit less?

- Does the person have concerns about what will happen to their personal information? It may help them if they have an explanation of who will see any information collected about them.

- For whose benefit is the technology being used? Are there problems with the technology for any other people?

- Are there any potential risks associated with the technology?

- Are there any alternatives to using the technology that might be more acceptable to the carer and the person living with dementia?

Take-home points

- ★ Technology has the potential to transform people's lives, and to keep people at home and independent for longer (Carers UK 2012).

While it can never replace the care and support provided by families we hope this chapter has demonstrated that it can complement this support.

* Technologies can help families in many different ways. It is important to find the technology that is right for you, addresses the challenges you face, and fits with your needs and circumstances. You should also consider the needs and wishes of the person living with dementia, if they will be affected by the technology.

* You do not need to invest in expensive, specialist technology. Simple equipment and technology can make a difference. Technology should make life easier, not add to stress or worry.

* Often the biggest barrier preventing families from using technology is simply a lack of knowledge about what is available. Ask health professionals, other people living with dementia and other carers what they recommend. Do your research – it can pay off!

* Dementia is a journey and people's needs and preferences often change over time. This can mean that technologies you have in place can become less useful or need to be replaced by something new. As new needs arise, revisit what solutions are available – remember this is a growing market and new things come out all the time.

* People can worry that technology can take over from contact with other people. However, technologies can allow carers to develop new relationships (for example via social forums) with people in similar situations. They can also provide new and helpful ways of spending time with, and keeping in touch with, the person with dementia they support.

* The Internet can be an incredible resource for families, as can online peer support communities, which offer a valuable source of support and shared learning. Remember though that no two people living with dementia (or carers) are alike and there are no 'one size fits all' solutions. Consider any information and advice in the context of your own circumstances, needs and values, as well as the situation of the person you support.

⋆ Technology has brought people together from across the world to support each other and share learning. This is incredibly powerful on a wider social level but also for individual carers – because sometimes the person who has been there for everyone else needs someone to be there for them.

Useful resources

Here are some places you can find more information about technology and dementia:

- Ask Sara: https://asksara.dlf.org.uk

- Living made easy: www.livingmadeeasy.org.uk

- AT Dementia: Assistive technology for people living with dementia: www.atdementia.org.uk

- Tunstall Healthcare UK YouTube channel: www.youtube.com/channel/UCqXujjbtyuTfhB1ViqP9uyg

- Alzheimer's Society UK website: www.alzheimers.org.uk and their page on assistive technology www.alzheimers.org.uk/info/20030/staying_independent/30/assistive_technology/4

- Carers UK, technology and equipment: www.carersuk.org/help-and-advice/technology-and-equipment

Acknowledgements

We would like to thank our CAREGIVERSPRO participants for sharing their helpful insights in what life is like supporting someone living with dementia.

Chapter 9

Technology for Organisations Supporting People with Dementia

Dr Julie Christie, *Region Manager UK and Europe, Dementia Centre, HammondCare, UK*

Professor Mary Marshall, *Senior Consultant, Dementia Centre, HammondCare, UK*

Introduction

Technology comes in many shapes and sizes. We use it to solve problems, to work creatively and to expand our reach and resources. It is humans, however, that drive the development of and use of technology and as such people are the most important part of any discussion on technological applications and solutions. People living with dementia are individuals, with their own stories, experiences, likes and dislikes. Organisations that provide high-quality care and support to older people and people with dementia know this and they continue this approach into their choices on technology use. Getting to know the person and ensuring that technology supports individual lifestyles and preferences is essential but not always easy. Technology is dynamic and advancing at a great speed. Organisations need to think about how it can be used cohesively and ethically, while continuing to deliver care and support in the present. In order to explore this in more detail this chapter will discuss the use of technology within an organisational context. We begin by introducing HammondCare, the organisation which features as our case study. We will then set the scene by highlighting the issues which face organisations that support people with dementia in their technology choices. In particular, we will discuss the different types of technology that are emerging in this space. We will then look at the ways in which technology can support organisational goals and values, how it can be used in innovative practice and the use of technology to support digital citizenship and engagement. Finally, we will consider how staff can be supported to use technology with confidence.

Introducing the organisation

HammondCare is an independent Christian charity specialising in dementia and aged care, palliative care, rehabilitation and older persons' mental health.[1] Regarded nationally and internationally as one of Australia's most innovative health and aged care providers, HammondCare offers hospital care, residential care and community services. It is both a major direct service provider and a significant indirect service provider in the form of a dementia centre.[2] The whole organisation supports approximately 17,000 people, employs over 3000 staff and works with approximately 800 volunteers across 63 service locations in Australia (HammondCare 2017). The Dementia Centre was founded in 1995; it works internationally to improve the lives of people with dementia and has a UK office with staff who work across the UK and Europe. HammondCare leads an industry partnership on behalf of the Australian government to provide Dementia Support Australia, a national support service which responds to referrals around understanding the behaviour of people living with dementia. This is achieved by telephone and where necessary by on-site visit. HammondCare is value-based with a clear vision which underpins all of its operations. It is passionate about improving quality of life for people in need.

Australia is big. It's really big. The total area of Australia is 7,692,024 square kilometres or 2,969,907 square miles.[3] To put this in context, if you were to sit Australia over a map of Europe, it would almost completely cover it. Australia has three main time zones: Australian Western Standard Time which is eight hours ahead of the time standard Coordinated Universal Time (UTC), Australian Central Standard Time (UTC+09:30), and Australian Eastern Standard Time

---

1   www.hammond.com.au
2   www.dementiacentre.com
3   thetruesize.com

(UTC+10:00). Time is regulated by the individual state governments, some of which also observe daylight saving time (DST). There is also a significant time difference between Australia and the UK (11 hours between London and Sydney, for example, outside British Summer Time). How does an organisation working across these vast geographical areas and time zones stay connected to its workforce and manage organisational objectives? Technology holds the key.

Technology use: What do we need to know?

The main issue in the implementation of technology in organisations that employ human service professionals is the danger of the erosion of human intimacy and, in turn, the organisation becoming less person focused and more process focused. Baldwin (2005) describes this as changing the contact between the person with dementia and the carer from person cared for/person caring towards user of technology/technology support worker. In his own exploration on the ethics of technology use with people with dementia, Baldwin referred to the work of Martin, Gutman and Hutton (1988) who identified four major types of technology:

- *Technologies of production*, which permit us to create, for example computer design software that allows us to build 3D spaces to visualise new care environments. Business technologies that support work practices would also be included here.

- *Technologies of sign systems* (sometimes referred to as language or communication), which allow us to recognise meanings and symbols. Examples would be the smartphone, video calls, chat apps, etc., and also call systems. This also includes educational technology such as software to support learning. Simulated presence would also feature in this category. This is where a family member, for example, might record a video for a person with dementia to play when they experience stress or distress. Simulated presence also applies to chatbots (computer programs which conduct conversations) and the developing use of robot companions.

- *Technologies of power*, which determine or monitor the conduct of individuals. These include assistive technologies such as the use of Global Positioning Systems (GPS) to track the movements of people with dementia, and pressure sensors. Some medical technologies also fall into this category, for example remote blood pressure devices, but also less obvious everyday examples such as fitness trackers.

• *Technologies of the self*, which support freedom of expression and action. These can be assistive technologies that promote independence, for example a 'digital personal assistant', and also entertainment technologies that support interests, leisure activities and fun, such as use of tablets in the creative arts or social media interest groups. Practical technology such as dynamic lighting systems would also fall into this category.

It is important to note that technologies can fall into more than one category. In the wrong hands an enabling technology can be used to restrict a person's freedom or choices. Vigilance is needed to ensure that technology and practice remain consistent with the organisation's values. Lynn *et al.* (2017) carried out a review of research into the use of electronic assistive technology within supported living environments for people with dementia. They also explored the extent to which people with dementia had been included in the research. They concluded that although there was a lack of evidence as to the types of intervention that are most effective, there is potential for a technology solution to be incorporated within a person-centred approach. It is useful to consider this alongside the technological categories listed above, as we present some examples from our case study organisation's use of technology to support its work with people living with dementia, and at the same time, retain a person-centred focus that promotes human experience and connection.

Technology to facilitate organisational values and goals

In order to meet the needs of the people with dementia, families and carers that an organisation supports, it must first find ways to communicate and sustain its values and standards with the workforce and to find ways to harness the knowledge and experience of staff in an asset-based approach. Technology can achieve this in a number of ways which we will now explore.

Connect and collaborate

Many organisations now provide a virtual 'meeting space' for staff through web-based collaborative programs such as SharePoint (Microsoft, created in 2001). Such platforms allow the organisation to develop an accessible means of storing content and managing documents online, which often replaces the need for corporate file servers. The content that is uploaded usually follows departmental structures such as human resources, information technology, and so on to meet the organisation's management, legal and policy requirements. An organisation can then create a web-based identity or an online office which is available at any time day or night and can be accessed from any location or while staff are on the move. In this way, information is centralised and vision, values, information and organisational communications can be facilitated. Teams also have their own subsites, so in the HammondCare example, the Dementia Centre has its own landing page within the larger shared space. SharePoint also contains team collaboration features including project scheduling, social collaboration, shared mailboxes, and project-related document storage and collaboration. Individual projects can have their own locked project sites, and this allows members of the team to work collaboratively from anywhere in the world. Information sharing and social networking are facilitated through regular video communications and chat sites. Staff are encouraged to ask questions and support each other with solutions to work-related issues, which fosters work-based relationships, recognises staff as assets and helps to develop a culture of peer support.

Staff also use cloud-based video conferencing facilities to facilitate discussions and meetings. Team meetings can then be joined remotely from different office sites and staff can also join individually. Diary scheduling takes account of the different time zones across Australia and the UK so that everyone joins the meeting at the right time from their particular location. Meetings are also recorded and uploaded onto team sites so that no one misses out. This ensures that staff feel valued and their contributions can be included.

Process and practice

Customer relationship management (CRM) systems are also used. These are cloud-based facilities which host case management and task management functions. In essence a CRM is a directory of contacts for your organisation. It is also a database of the people who use an organisation's services. Related documents such as assessments and reports can be filed and tasks associated with each person can be scheduled, managed and recorded. Taking the example of Dementia Support Australia, all referrals to this service are recorded on a CRM system which forms the client database. In addition a robust telephone system is required that can deal efficiently with practicalities such as call volume and the call purpose of responding to people in need of support. To this end part of the process also has to be about finding space within the system to talk to people and hear about the difficulties that they are experiencing. The system, therefore, routes call traffic 24 hours a day to the next available consultant in order that all calls are responded to within a target of 20 seconds. Referrals can also be made using a web referral system. Data analysis is built into the process in order that the reasons for referral, activities, outputs and outcomes can be better understood, but also to map geographical patterns of activity.

Training, learning and CPD

A culture of learning can be promoted through virtual knowledge clusters and webinars. These approaches utilise cloud-based technology in order to facilitate learning, peer support and research activities. These can be used to complement more traditional learning formats.

Virtual reality (VR) refers to computer-generated immersive and interactive experiences. Or more simply, while wearing a headset a person can enter a real or imaginary setting and interact with this new environment, moving freely around and experiencing sights, sounds and other sensory experiences. Early adopters of VR in practice and research found that they were limited by technology. For example, screens and computers were fixed, meaning that people needed to travel to a specific place for a limited session. VR in its current form, however, has developed alongside new technologies in gaming and smartphones, combining interactive gaming experiences with accessibility and mobility. Improvements in software and hardware mean that more sophisticated programs and a more immersive sense of reality can be achieved with headsets that are not tethered to a computer or location.

This opens up the potential use of VR to people in a whole range of settings.

The Virtual Reality Empathy Platform (VR-EP) is a groundbreaking virtual reality platform, developed with insights and expertise from HammondCare Dementia Centre in partnership with two Scottish companies – Aitken Turnbull Architects and Wireframe Immersive.[4] Described in the *Royal Institute of British Architects Journal* as 'cutting edge immersive software designed to help architects improve the lives of people living with dementia' (Cousins 2017), this platform can guide designers and builders in developing environments for people living with dementia. Through this device, we can explore potential environments as a person with dementia, sharing daily sensory challenges. For example, a person with dementia might perceive patterns on a carpet to be moving, or toilets might seem to disappear if they are in an all-white bathroom. Similarly, from an acoustic perspective you might find that the experience of background noise can be distracting, stressful or overwhelming. While these environmental experiences can be explained to architects, designers and care staff it is quite another thing to experience the environment for yourself as a person with dementia might. This product can also be used to replicate proposed designs, such as a new care home, as a virtual environment, and allow commissioners to experience and test out dementia-inclusive design elements, as a person with dementia, before committing to build. The VR-EP simulates changes associated with the ageing eye and is built on a case study of a specific person with dementia, the fictional Grace McDonald. It is anticipated that through this combination of immersive story and environment, new learning experiences could be generated for care staff, and new learning outcomes that can help inform dementia education, knowledge and skills for care sector staff could be realised.

Technology that supports innovative practice

As illustrated in the above example, innovation and technology go hand in hand; however, it can be easy for the excitement of new technology to take precedence over the principles of good dementia practice. The use of technology should support and complement existing evidence-based practice. The other chapters in this book cover in detail

---

4   http://vr-ep.com

technology that supports people with dementia as they live their lives and the ethical considerations in their use. Here, we will focus on the use of technology from an organisational perspective.

'If you meet one person with dementia, you have met one person with dementia' reminds us that although we talk about 'people' with dementia, we are in fact working to support many unique 'persons' who have a range of individual needs and preferences for which we have to design services. People with dementia have unique backgrounds and will differ in what environmental and technological features make them feel comfortable and empowered. Ageing and age also have to play a factor. People with dementia vary in the era from which they are now making sense of the world. Each person can vary greatly in terms of physical, sensory and cognitive impairments. Most care settings have people aged between 80 and 100 years, and sometimes much younger people as well, living in group settings. And importantly, we are all different because of the lives we have led and our own unique experiences. Technology, like any other aspect of care, has to take all of this into account.

Technology used by staff in their work with people with dementia

Technology is widely used in direct care provision. The residential provision of HammondCare is delivered in small, domestic, carefully designed cottages. Their design promotes independence and wayfinding while at the same time allowing unobtrusive and respectful surveillance. As far as technology is concerned, in any cottage you would find:

- Technology that monitors a person's routine in order to establish a baseline or pattern of behaviour. Thereafter, staff are only alerted by exception. This technology includes motion sensors and infrared door sensors.

- Technology to address identified issues, for example fall detectors for anyone at risk of falling, pressure sensors on beds and floor, use of GPS and door sensors for anyone assessed as at risk of being lost.

- A silent nurse call system which is linked to individual staff pagers. In previous years, nurse call systems with audible beeps and blinking lights were prevalent; however, these are now considered as reinforcing institutional environments and detracting from the priority that a care home is first and foremost a person's home. They also contribute to acoustic intrusion and sensory overload.

- Environmental monitoring: devices which contribute to wellbeing by ensuring optimum lighting and noise levels and thermal comfort. Acoustic intrusion devices such as 'yacker trackers' show staff the level of decibels in any situation using a traffic light system and can help to reduce noise levels significantly.

The important factor in all of this, however, is that the technology supports the person to live as independently as possible. Technology use, therefore, has to be built around knowledge of each individual. So, for example, if we know that someone likes to get out of bed during the night when they are unable to sleep, the motion detectors being activated won't necessarily result in nurse intrusion. Technology can then support privacy and individual lifestyles instead of being used to regiment behaviour and routine. The focus of the nurse call system is to allow residents (and staff) to seek assistance if and when they need it but to continue their day-to-day life without interruption. A software interface supports managers to edit alert settings and run reports.

Wearable technology, which is technology that can be worn as an accessory, has grown in popularity in the recent past. The availability of this store-purchased tech has seen it move from the realms of professional athletes to ordinary people who are interested in monitoring their own fitness and health. The accessories vary in terms of intrusiveness; by this we mean issues of both privacy and comfort. For example, wearable tech includes bracelets and watches, which many people wear already, through to heart-monitoring chest straps. Periods of activity and inactivity and sleep quality can also be recorded. Records can be kept locally on the device or updated to cloud storage. It is, therefore, important that when such technology is used the person understands what it will record, in what ways, where their information will be stored, who will have access to the information and how the information could be used. There are currently pilots looking at the use of such technology to inform our understanding of frailty, to enable self-management programmes and to support assessments of people with dementia. It is not, of course, straightforward since some people with dementia will be unable to consent, and some may be unwilling to wear a strange device.

Case study 9.1 Alice's story

Mrs Alice Veitch moved to Sydney to be near her daughter but until she was 75 years old, she had lived on a sheep station near a small town, well south of Canberra. She and her husband took over from her father when he died so she had never lived anywhere else. She was an active member of the local church and most of her social life centred on church activities.

She had a small flat in Sydney but recently her dementia progressed to such an extent that she was unable to remain there and moved into a HammondCare cottage. She has been there two months and is very restless. It has proved difficult to monitor her routine in any way, which means that staff have to keep an eye on her, and at night they respond to the sensors in her room whenever she shows signs of getting out of bed. She is very unsteady on her feet and is likely to fall if not assisted.

Mrs Veitch can be diverted using a book of photographs of her previous property or, using Google Earth, by looking at the locality. She also very much enjoys the services from the local church which are live-streamed onto her iPad. For short periods she enjoys familiar hymns on her personal playlist. She is more relaxed on her own outside. Staff are considering whether her restlessness might be related to the extent of activity and noise in the cottage, since Mrs Veitch has led a quiet life on her own for many years. They are also using 'pain check' to assess the possibility that she is experiencing pain which she cannot express.

Nadya Siddiqui is a member of the night staff. She has consulted Mrs Veitch's daughter about her early morning routine since she has become aware that Mrs Veitch wakes before first light and is particularly agitated. She now takes Mrs Veitch through to the kitchen where they make a cup of coffee and then sit at the door to the outside watching the sun come up. Nadya can be alerted to any other resident needing assistance because there will be a silent alert on her pager if someone acts outside their normal routine. Nadya is thus able to focus on being in the present with Mrs Veitch, enabling her to start the day with a sense of calm.

Pain assessment and management

A pain recognition app that assesses pain levels in people with dementia is set to speed up the diagnosis and treatment of pain. The new app, called PainChek™, has specific application for people with dementia who have challenges with verbal communication to improve their quality of lives. The app uses artificial intelligence and smartphone technology to visually analyse facial expressions, assess pain levels in real time and update cloud-based medical records. An outcome of dementia can be a loss of ability to communicate and when that person is in pain it is sometimes displayed in frustration or behaviour that is out of character. As a result, pain for people living with dementia may often go undetected or under-treated. This technology helps staff to quickly identify if a person is in pain.

Virtual reality for the treatment of pain has been around for some time. However, it has been used primarily in the acute pain setting. For example, a virtual reality 'game' called SnowWorld allows people with pain after severe burns to travel and interact with a world of snow and ice. This is basically a form of distraction and has now been used in other settings to reduce the pain of short-term procedures and operations. It is only more recently that there has been interest in treating chronic pain with VR. There is now evidence that chronic pain is linked to changes in the brain, particularly in scenarios like amputation or spinal cord injury. It is believed that these changes occur because the brain no longer gets the normal visual and sensory cues from the missing limb or below the spinal cord injury, and the brain tries to reorganise to accommodate. Unfortunately, these brain changes appear to be linked to pain. VR can be used to create an environment where people can interact with each other and the virtual world, and have a strong impression that they can move their missing limb, and it is believed that this may reverse the brain changes that cause the pain. The research in this area is very young but there are some promising signs that it may be a useful and effective new approach. The increased accessibility of VR means that people with chronic pain can be treated frequently because they can use a VR more regularly, either on a daily basis or when the pain is severe. It also opens up the possibility of providing another effective non-medication option for people who are trying to keep medication use to a minimum to avoid side effects and have few other options. However, the use of virtual reality by people with dementia is still an under-researched area.

Technology, citizenship and engagement

Technology has the potential to facilitate engagement on a number of levels. The accessibility of phones and tablets means that more people than ever before are able to stay connected to friends and family from anywhere in the world. Issues of digital citizenship and social media use with respect to people living with dementia who are in receipt of care are now coming to the fore. *Digital citizen* refers to a person utilising information technology in order to engage in society, politics and government participation. It is, therefore, argued that this aspect of life is as important as any other, as it is integral to societal participation and being part of a larger community. Increasingly, more people than ever are using social media, so this is an issue that cannot be ignored. However, many care homes, unlike HammondCare, do not have open WiFi for residents. This is despite there being readily available WiFi in public spaces and even on public transport.

Technology can also support interaction with the arts. Music is used extensively in HammondCare residential care in New South Wales and Victoria, Australia, by care staff, in conjunction with family, friends and volunteers. The organisation has implemented a three-pronged approach to music engagement: individualised music, group participatory music and creative expressive music making. There is not one single approach to music in dementia care which is best. Individualised and tailored music has been found to leverage benefits of deep emotional connection to reduce pain, alleviate anxiety and address distressed behaviours. Group participatory music can foster socialisation, belonging, integration and the sense of community. Creative expressive music making gives 'voice' and expression to people who may not be able to speak up in conversation and nurtures enablement, creativity, choice and agency. This diverse approach to music engagement enables those supporting or searching for ways to connect to a person living with dementia to use music in a way that is flexible and responsive, centred on individual need. Unit costs for individualised, tailored music or instruments for expressive creation can be quantified by measures such as the cost of the equipment and the music, and the administrative cost for set-up and distribution. A rough estimate incorporating headphones, a music storage device, music resources, storage, etc. in an individualised music 'kit' is around £92–£123 ($150–200 AUD), contingent on the scale of music resources in the organisation. However, the flexible, responsive and individualised approach of music engagement means that the time and labour of care staff is not a discrete measure.

While no distinct cost-benefit analyses have been conducted, music engagement has been used successfully in specific response to people who feel distressed. Targeted music interventions to reduce agitation triggered by visitors to the home and bathing, and distressed behaviours, have been used in high-care and behaviour-specialist care settings. The impact of individualised music as an intervention to reduce severely distressed behaviour has emerged as profound, with the advantage of being inexpensive and non-pharmacological, i.e. without side effects or interactions with other medications, which technology can support.

Supporting staff to use technology with confidence

It is also important to remember that organisations are made up of in-dividuals with varying interest, skills and knowledge on technology and its applications. All workplaces use technology to varying degrees and many of us have learnt the skills and processes needed as new digital solutions have been adopted. However, the pace of change is now such that organisations have to commit learning space and time to ensuring that their workforce are supported in their use of technology. We would recommend that organisations have a position statement on their use of technology alongside organisational guides. Technology champions within the workplace over and above IT teams (which focus more on installation, maintenance and upgrades) also help to embed new technologies or to support employees who are anxious about new technology. Tech mentors can also be useful. Organisations need to ensure that issues of ethical use of technology and the data generated through use (for example, how will data be stored, handled and destroyed?) alongside the need for consent and the process for obtaining this are addressed. As with all interventions evaluation is essential. With regard to technology this should include what we use, the impact of use and the experience of the user; however, this is often overlooked. In this way a system of learning and feedback can be established to ensure that person-focused values remain at the heart of our practice.

Take-home points

Working closely with people living with dementia and their families is a privilege. High-quality dementia care and support needs to be delivered by skilled, compassionate staff. Technology is now part of the toolkit to help us support people with dementia as they live their lives. Learning about each person and their everyday lives can help us in our technology choices, ranging from social media and entertainment devices through to medical devices and telecare options. Ethical practice requires us to reflect on the balance between control and empowerment, and between risk enablement and the need to help people to remain safe and well.

Organisations therefore should encourage staff to think about:

* This particular person and their life.

* What technology to use and when to use it.

* Can you use this technology in this situation, from an organisational perspective, taking into account costs and practicalities?

* Should you use technology in this situation?

* In what ways will it support this person?

* In what ways will it support my work and values?

* What will this technology replace?

* What will I lose if I use this technology?

In particular the 'What will I lose?' question can often take staff by surprise. For example, the use of some devices can reduce the amount of face-to-face interaction with the person that you are working with; however, if it frees up your workforce for more meaningful, less institutional engagement at other times this might be preferable. If, instead, it removes the need for any meaningful interaction with the person concerned the reasons for use might need more considered thought, as it could reveal deeper issues in the organisation's values and respect for people with dementia.

In summary, technology should be used to add value to our strategies, processes and procedures as part of a connected, cohesive system. At all times the person with dementia, their needs and lifestyle preferences should be at the heart of decisions on use. Much like good design, good use of technology goes largely unnoticed as it fits seamlessly into the person's life. Supporting staff in digital literacy alongside value-based practice will ensure that the organisation, the workforce and the people who use the services that we provide can move forward with confidence together, no matter what technological updates the future holds.

Chapter 10

Dementia-Friendly Future

Dr Stephen Czarnuch, *Assistant Professor,*
Department of Electrical and Computer Engineering/Discipline of
Emergency Medicine, Memorial University, Newfoundland, Canada

Professor Arlene Astell, *Professor of Neurocognitive Disorders,*
University of Reading, UK and Research Chair in Dementia,
Ontario Shores Centre for Mental Health Sciences, Canada

Introduction

The concept of 'dementia friendliness' emerged in Japan in the 1990s, where cities such as Uji highlighted that people who engaged with a community support network fared better and lived longer in the community. From this early work an international concept emerged, defined by Alzheimer's Disease International as 'a place or culture in which people with dementia and their carers are empowered, supported and included in society, understand their rights and recognise their full potential' (Alzheimer's Disease International n.d.). A list of global dementia-friendly initiatives can be found on their website.[1] In the UK, examples include dementia-friendly train stations (e.g. Durham, Darlington), towns (e.g. Purley; Watts 2017) and the Dementia Friends programme (Department of Health and Social Care 2012).

Along with these community-based and environmental initiatives, what might be the role of technology in a dementia-friendly future? Throughout this book, we have considered past and current technology innovations, and the roles they may play in research, treatment and care for people with dementia and their caregivers. We have seen that technological innovations in dementia have been going in parallel with basic science for almost 40 years, addressing the many and complex

---

1   www.alz.co.uk/dementia-friendly-communities/case-studies

challenges people with dementia face (Chapter 1). We have examined the best ways to understand the needs of people with dementia for technology and how to support them to use it (Chapter 2) and considered some of the main ethical challenges in the design, uptake and use of technologies in dementia (Chapter 3). We have considered the wide range of technologies to support people at home (Chapter 4) and when they go out (Chapter 5), as well as the range of leisure pursuits technology can support (Chapter 6). We have heard the experiences of people living with dementia in how they make decisions and use technology in their everyday lives (Chapter 7). We have also examined technology available to support family caregivers (Chapter 8) and organisations supporting people who are living with dementia (Chapter 9). In this final chapter we consider the potential future of technology innovations in dementia, and specifically the future of technology for making the world dementia friendly, to support people to live well with dementia.

Potential future technology innovations in dementia

As we have shown throughout this book, technology has the potential to become pervasive in the lives of people with dementia and their caregivers in novel and exciting ways. Innovations are always under development to help in and out of the home, in communities and throughout society, supporting, educating and promoting life and healthy living. On the horizon of development are many new and exciting novel approaches that will potentially guide the future of dementia. Some of these developments have the potential to revolutionise dementia research, treatment and care. Some may even become disruptive technologies or disruptive innovations – technologies or innovations that will transform current practices by displacing or replacing the way we currently do things. Looking to the future of technology innovations in dementia in this context, we now consider artificial intelligence in general and specifically machine learning, big data and data mining, and cloud computing and the Internet of Things as potential disruptive technologies in dementia.

Artificial intelligence

Artificial intelligence (AI) is a controversial topic, specifically with respect to what is actually considered AI. Meriam-Webster broadly defines AI as: '1 a branch of computer science dealing with the simulation of intelligent behavior in computers'; and '2 the capability of a machine to imitate intelligent human behavior' (Merriam-Webster 2018). These definitions are intentionally and accurately broad. Notably, as the field of AI develops and tasks that were once computationally challenging become possible, the idea of what the term 'intelligent' means also evolves – known as the AI effect (Hofstadter 1979). This dynamic nature of AI was adeptly summarised in the 1970s by Larry Tesler, who was credited as foreseeing that 'AI is whatever hasn't been done yet' (Hofstadter 1979, p.597), a quote that he later corrected to be 'Intelligence is whatever machines haven't done yet' (Tesler 2018). In this context, AI applications have seen significant growth and potential in dementia research and treatment, particularly spurred on by advances in computers and computational methods. Under this broad understanding of what AI means, we now consider the role of AI in the future of dementia. Specifically, we consider one of the more novel and emergent area of research and application in dementia using AI: the diagnosis of dementia using machine learning.

Diagnosis of dementia and disease progression using machine learning

Diagnosing dementia can be complicated, involving an assortment of tests and multifaceted assessments, and is generally performed by a doctor or specialist such as a psychiatrist, neurologist or gerontologist. Though largely reliable for diagnosis, the current process is costly and time consuming, and some even argue unsustainable, given the projected increases in dementia globally. Accordingly, the early, accurate, repeatable, portable and cost-effective assessment of dementia has economic and personal significance. In recent years, various machine learning (ML) approaches have seen increasing application to the diagnosis of dementia.

The term 'machine learning' is credited to the work of Samuel (1959) and his attempt to program a machine that could learn from experience and 'play a better game of checkers than can be played by the person who wrote the program' (p.210). Since then, a more widely adopted explanation of machine learning, paraphrased for simplicity, is a computer program that learns from experience with respect to a task and performance measure, such that its performance in the task, assessed by the measure, improves with experience (Mitchell 1997). In dementia technologies, perhaps the most common ML approaches are used with imaging data for diagnosis and disease progression (Dallora *et al.* 2017), such as amyloid PET imaging (e.g. Cabral *et al.* 2015; Mathotaarachchi *et al.* 2017), MR imaging (e.g. Cheng *et al.* 2015; Liu *et al.* 2014), and a combination of PET and MR imaging (e.g. Liu *et al.* 2014). Diagnosis and progression approaches that do not use imaging data generally focus on demographical data and cognitive measures (e.g. Bhagyashree *et al.* 2017; Seixas *et al.* 2014; Tandon, Adak and Kaye 2006), or in some more recent studies utilise novel linguistic analysis (e.g. Fraser, Meltzer and Rudzicz 2016; König *et al.* 2015b). Other approaches utilise a synthesis of imaging and non-imaging data to include as many potential predictive factors as possible at the cost of increased complexity (e.g. Cui *et al.* 2011; Ye *et al.* 2012). Regardless of the data sources used, current ML approaches are arguably closest to clinical application in both the diagnosis of dementia and the evaluation of disease progression over time. As more data become available and ML approaches continue to develop, this area of research and application will surely continue to flourish. Indeed, data collection and storage has exploded recently, leading not only to more data for such ML approaches, but also to new opportunities related to these large data sets themselves, known as 'big data'.

Big data and data mining

Big data, in comparison to more conventional data sets, is a concept that emerged in the early 2000s in response to the sheer amount of data being collected and stored globally, and the potential to analyse these data. Like artificial intelligence, the term 'big data' has become widely used without a formal definition (Schroeder 2014), but rather with many broad and varying conceptualisations. Perhaps the most widely accepted definition of big data identifies three key data features: volume (huge amounts), velocity (pressure for fast, or real-time, processing) and variety (heterogeneity of data and sources). Notably, big data is also characterised by challenges with data collection, storage, analysis and sharing (among others) as well as privacy and security, which in most contexts are unique issues compared to more traditional data sets. Big data approaches are increasingly seeing application to complex diseases like dementia (Hofmann-Apitius 2015), particularly because of the large volume and variety of the data currently associated with dementia, collected from both research and practice across many disciplines. Additionally, there are still significant opportunities for contributing to advances in treatments for dementia beyond traditional research approaches, which currently show limited effectiveness at finding a cure. This is exemplified by the fact that there are no drugs currently on the market to cure dementia or stop progression (Alzheimer's Association 2017), and no new drugs proposed in over a decade (Richards 2017). This situation is a popular scenario for the application of big data research in biomedicine in general, as well as dementia specifically (Doubal *et al.* 2017; Hofmann-Apitius 2015).

The response to the potential for big data in dementia treatment and research has been felt both globally and locally. For example, in 2013 the G8 health ministers mandated the Organisation for Economic Co-operation and Development to explore the use of big data in dementia research following the G8 Global Dementia Summit (University of Oxford for the Oxford Internet Institute 2014). The Big Data for Advancing Dementia Research project was initiated, resulting in a formal report (Deetjen, Meyer and Schroeder 2015) presented to the first World Health Organization Ministerial Conference on Global Action Against Dementia in Geneva in 2015. Findings suggested that big data had the potential to accelerate dementia research and technology development, helping recognise factors that contribute to dementia, identifying individuals with dementia earlier, promoting better support for dementia care, and creating new analysis methods (e.g. data mining) that may result in new research opportunities. A recent commentary on the use of big data in dementia research further supported, among other issues, the importance of data mining on the future of dementia research (Hofmann-Apitius 2015). Accordingly, we now briefly consider what data mining is, and present some emerging trends in this new field of dementia research.

Data mining is defined as 'the science of extracting useful knowledge from…huge data repositories' (Chakrabarti *et al.* 2006, p.1). Of course, in this context huge data repositories are synonymous with big data. As data collection increasingly contributes to big data sets of dementia-related data, new opportunities to process those data continue to appear. For example, data mining recently has been used with large, pre-existing data registries and health records to investigate co-morbidities with dementia and other diseases (Chen, Yang and Lee 2016; Fereshtehnejad *et al.* 2014) and to predict five-year life expectancy (Mathias *et al.* 2013). Promising results by these and other studies support the suggestion that big data and data mining techniques are definitely going to be a part of the future of dementia research. Indeed, dementia research stands to benefit from advances in modern computers and computing, where 'for the first time in history we not only have volumes of the right data but we also have the means to be able to analyse it' (Richards 2017). The power of big data and data mining partially comes from individual researchers and clinicians sharing and making accessible their big data sets and analytical approaches to other individual researchers and clinicians, but also through contributing globally as a collective. This need for global accessibility and utilisation has resulted in the emergence of new forms of digital connection, computing and storage, generally connected to the nebulous concept of 'the cloud'. In this context, the cloud simply refers to digital services that run through the Internet, rather than on a local computer.

Cloud computing and the Internet of Things

Cloud computing is a technology paradigm in which devices have pervasive and universal access to shared, and generally online, computing resources. The concept of cloud computing actually dates back to the 1960s, but the modern understanding of cloud computing via the Internet was brought to mass popularity in 2006 via the release of the Elastic Compute Cloud by Amazon (Amazon Web Services 2006), followed by Microsoft's Windows Azure in 2010 (eventually renamed Microsoft Azure; Microsoft 2010), and Google Compute Engine in 2013 (Google 2013). Ultimately, the purpose of these cloud computing platforms is to allow any potential user to focus on their application through transparent and simple access to these technologies without significant skill and expertise in the actual technologies. Cloud computing allows dementia researchers and practitioners the ability to utilise powerful computing resources without the need for specialised computing backgrounds. The result is that research is less expensive and faster to produce results. For these reasons, many novel research projects investigating cloud-based solutions to dementia care, treatment and diagnosis have emerged recently. Examples of these include supporting ageing in place and activity monitoring (Li *et al.* 2016; Mihailidis 2017), providing location tracking (Yaw-Jen, Heng-Shuen and Mei-Ju 2015) and supporting the neuroimaging analysis efforts of dementia researchers and practitioners (Shen, Kennedy and Preuss 2013).

In dementia research, a concept related to cloud computing is the Internet of Things (IoT). The IoT, as the name suggests, is the connection of 'things' such as medical devices and health records via networks like the Internet. Practically speaking, the IoT facilitates the connection of real things in the real world to computer systems, providing data to such systems more easily, efficiently and economically. Notably, and relevant to dementia research, some argue that the IoT concept supports a broader range of 'things' than simply electronic devices, generalising to software, hardware and data, but also including services (Noto La Diega and Walden 2016). The IoT is relatively new in the field of dementia research specifically, but has already seen broad application to both the healthcare and pharmaceutical industries, as well as assisted living research (Dimitrioglou, Kardaras and Barbounaki 2017). In dementia, the IoT has largely focused on the actual technical connection of devices (e.g. Del Campo *et al.* 2016; Shin, Shin and Shin 2014). Still, more recently the IoT has been integrated into the early phases of full healthcare integration (Enshaeifar *et al.* 2018), confirming its potential in the future of dementia research and care.

Informed design: Science, technology and society

In this chapter, we have considered some current technology innovations in dementia that may impact the future of dementia treatment and research. Now, we consider some methodological factors that may impact technology innovations in dementia in the future, with a specific focus on research into technologies. Central to the future of technologies for dementia is that technology and society do not exist independently from each other. Historically, technology has played a significant role in shaping society, and conversely society has shaped the development and acceptance of technology. The dependence and co-construction of society and technology on each other is well documented, reaching back to the beginning of human existence. The academic study of the synergistic and reciprocal relationship between society and technology emerged as an interdisciplinary programme formally in the 1970s. Called Science and Technology Studies, hundreds of programmes now exist worldwide (STS Wiki 2010). Most notable and relevant in a modern context is the recent development of digital technologies like computers and the Internet, which have become pervasive in our lives and in society in general (Ruckriem 2009). The study of science and technology includes how they impact many facets of society, including their ethical, economic, cultural and future impact (e.g. University of Alberta 2017).

Though the field of science and technology studies is relatively new, and definitions of what is included in the field vary, we highlight some main themes related to the future of dementia research: (1) who participates in technology research and how; (2) who the stakeholders are in decision making regarding technologies; (3) how risk and safety are assessed and enforced; (4) how information is shared between researchers and the public; and (5) how research funding priorities are allocated (President and Fellows of Harvard College 2017). Specifically, we now consider how multidisciplinary and interdisciplinary teams have emerged to address the first two themes regarding participants in technology research. We then discuss how user-centred design philosophies may address the third theme, including not only risk and safety, but also the appropriateness and efficacy of technologies for dementia. We then consider citizen science as a potential future direction for dementia research that will help address the theme regarding the relationship between researchers and the public, and as a means of extending the capabilities of research teams. Finally, we discuss the fifth theme, the future of funding for technology research for dementia.

Multidisciplinary technology research teams

The trajectory of dementia, as well as personal experiences with dementia, are diverse and varied, both for people with dementia and their caregivers. Furthermore, if we look around the globe, we see that resources available to treat and support dementia vary substantially at the national, regional and individual level. Accordingly, since technology for dementia doesn't exist only in the realm of natural sciences, there is a growing recognition of the need to include multidisciplinary research teams with members holding different areas of expertise to reflect this diversity and variety in neurological disorder research in general (e.g. Quaglio *et al.* 2017), and dementia research specifically (Alzheimer's Research UK 2012; Marjanovic *et al.* 2016; Stuss *et al.* 2015). Notably, the importance of multidisciplinary teams extends beyond research into technology (applications, devices) through to clinical practice and dementia care (Grand, Caspar and MacDonald 2011; Schols and Kardol 2017).

Multidisciplinary research teams are generally considered to be teams composed of researchers with different backgrounds. Members of multidisciplinary dementia research teams may include researchers from diverse fields such as psychology, engineering, computer science, sociology, gerontology, dentistry, medicine, nursing, pharmacy, social work and neurology (e.g. Alm *et al.* 2007; Czarnuch *et al.* 2013; Tan *et al.* 2017; van Kooten *et al.* 2015). However, multidisciplinary teams can also include people with dementia and their formal or informal caregivers, and other stakeholders such as healthcare administrators and policy decision makers. The role of participants other than researchers can also vary in multidisciplinary teams. Traditionally, family caregivers have been asked to act as a proxy for people with dementia, who for many years were not considered able to participate independently. However, more recent approaches have directly involved people with dementia in the research (e.g. Astell *et al.* 2009) while others focus on caregivers as the research population (e.g. Czarnuch, Ricciardelli and Mihailidis 2016). Other multidisciplinary teams include patients and caregivers directly as researchers, engaging in peer research (see Di Lorito *et al.* 2017 for a review). Regardless of the composition of the team or the specific role of the members, undoubtedly multidisciplinary teams will be an important component of the future of dementia research (Stuss *et al.* 2015), improving research quality and leading to better outcomes (Lepore *et al.* 2017; Morgan *et al.* 2014), and giving voice to those stakeholders who are most impacted by dementia – people with dementia, family caregivers and healthcare providers. Including key stakeholders in the design process is critical to helping ensure the acceptance and adoption of technology innovations. Accordingly, user-centred design has emerged as a development philosophy in dementia research to help ensure that technology users' needs are ultimately met.

User-centred design

The concept of user-centred design in dementia research mandates that technological interventions are developed to accommodate the user, rather than requiring the user to change to accommodate the technology. This process requires that prototypes are developed and evaluated against design targets throughout the design process, then re-developed and re-evaluated repeatedly, eventually culminating in real-world trials with real users. Accordingly, design teams must include people with dementia and their caregivers, or other stakeholders, as active members of all stages of design and development, rather than just during evaluations (Czarnuch and Mihailidis 2011). Implementing a user-centred design philosophy involves multiple iterative stages (Bharucha *et al.* 2009). The process generally begins with an unbiased assessment with the users of their needs, preferences, behaviours, environmental and social conditions, support networks, goals or outcomes, risks and safety requirements, and any other factors relevant to a new technology. These details provide the overall context of use for introduction and use of the technology.

Next, this context, which in many cases is quite complex and multifaceted, is translated into specific design criteria for the technology, through formal design approaches involving the entire multidisciplinary research team. These design criteria are used to develop functional prototypes that are evaluated against the technical design criteria and against the contextual criteria. Initially, evaluations are often conducted in controlled locations with ideal conditions (e.g. design laboratories), but eventually progress to real-world environments with real users in real scenarios. Through an iterative design loop, evaluation outcomes are used both to refine the technical design criteria, and to inform the development of new prototypes, eventually converging on solutions that are likely to be accepted and adopted into use. In dementia technology research, user-centred design has seen varied application over the past decade. For example, technology-focused dementia projects have covered a wide range of goals, including developing assistive technologies (e.g. Thorpe *et al.* 2016), enhancing quality of life (e.g. Müller-Rakow and Flechtner 2017), supporting caregivers (e.g. Cristancho-Lacroix *et al.* 2014), and creating infrastructure and information-sharing systems for use by dementia clinicians (e.g. Smaradottir *et al.* 2015) to name a few. The power of user-centred design is clear, as is the usefulness and effectiveness of multidisciplinary teams towards developing useful and efficacious technologies. However, a research team is naturally limited to a functional size. Additionally, research teams are limited in both space and time, based on the location of the team members and the period in which the team is collaborating. Accordingly, considering the future of dementia innovation, we now turn to the idea of citizen science – a method of transcending limitations with research across time and space, while simultaneously engaging the public in research.

Citizen science

The idea that the public can contribute to science and research emerged as a mainstream concept in the mid-1990s. Formally termed 'citizen science', the idea has two predominant motivations or purposes. The first, and most common motivation, is that many complex problems require substantial amounts of data such that it is not feasible, practical or economical for a small group of scientists to collect (Bonney *et al.* 2009). For these types of projects and problems, the general public can serve as a contributor to a public database of information. This type of citizen science has had great success with projects like bird tracking (e.g. Audubon and Cornell Lab of Ornithology 2017[2]), meteor observation (e.g. American Meteor Society Ltd 2017[3]) and climate monitoring (e.g. Alaska Native Tribal Health Consortium (ANTHC) 2016). Notably, this type of citizen science is subject to potentially biased or erroneous data since the collection is often completed by the public who do not, in general, have proper research training (Thelen and Thiet 2008). Accordingly, many current citizen science projects are coordinated or supervised by researchers and scientists, leading to the definition of 'scientific work undertaken by members of the general public, often in collaboration with or under the direction of professional scientists and scientific institutions' (OED Online 2017).

The second, and less common, motivation behind citizen science is to ensure that science and research are conducted in an open and transparent manner (Riesch and Potter 2013) according to the early ideas of Alan Irwin (1995). In this way, both the public and scientists

---

2   http://ebird.org/content/ebird
3   www.amsmeteors.org

hold an equal role in the research across the spectrum, including the identification of relevant needs, knowledge and information generation, and dissemination (Hemment, Ellis and Wynne 2011; Riesch and Potter 2013). Notably, although both of these conceptualisations of citizen science exist, they are indeed different and are generally exercised independent of one another. In rare cases, a blended fusion of both forms of citizen science is realised (e.g. Forestry Commission 2011), though some would argue that this fused approach is undertheorised (Riesch and Potter 2013).

Dementia is a complicated syndrome, having a significant impact on people with dementia, their caregivers and the healthcare systems globally. For this reason, both forms of citizen science have begun to emerge as a means of contributing to the research and treatment of dementia. For example, in the UK a large-scale citizen science project has emerged to support research on dementia by providing a strong voice to those who live with dementia and their caregivers (Ctrl Group 2017). This project, called Dementia Citizens, takes a multifaceted approach to citizen science following the ideals of both Irwin (1995) and Bonney (Bonney *et al.* 2009). People with dementia and their caregivers are empowered to share and learn, while helping contribute real-world data to various ongoing studies. Other studies follow Bonney's concept of citizen science more directly, using the general public for data collection (e.g. Morgan 2016) or data analysis assistance (e.g. EyesOnALZ[4]). Still others follow Irwin's concept, focusing on making dementia resources, research and information more readily available to the public (e.g. MOPEAD 2016). However, regardless of the motivation, strength in numbers and the importance of public engagement will undoubtedly result in more citizen science projects emerging in the near future to help contribute to dementia research and treatment.

Funding and support for technology for dementia

Individual researchers and research teams have sought a cure for dementia for decades, though in more recent years a united global effort to fight Alzheimer's disease and other forms of dementia has emerged (e.g. World Health Organization 2017). This international reaction has largely come

---

4   http://hcjournal.org/wecurealz

about in response to the increasing prevalence of dementia globally, and its associated impact on social, economic, political and healthcare systems (Alzheimer's Disease International 2015). Initial efforts sought a cure for dementia, and a substantial amount of investment was allocated to projects that ultimately failed to develop of any drugs to treat dementia. Between 1998 and 2014, a total of 123 different drugs were developed to treat Alzheimer's disease alone, without a single successful drug making it to market (PhRMA 2015). Much of the funding for these unsuccessful attempts at a cure was provided by drug companies, though some governments and private organisations also provided investment into a cure. During that same period, only four new drugs were approved to treat the symptoms of the disease. This lack of success has resulted in a 'funding fatigue', whereby drug companies and donors are reluctant to fund further research out of concern of failure and lack of return on investment (Rubinstein *et al.* 2015, p.28). The result is that researchers and academics are increasingly forced to compete for funding for dementia research from decreasing pools of money. Funding for dementia technology research, which accounts for only a fraction of the total funding pool that is largely supportive of drug development, has resultantly become even more sparse and competitive.

Largely motivated by the increasing recognition that dementia is a global issue, funding for dementia research in general is again increasing, and opportunities specifically focused on innovative dementia research are also emerging. For example, the Dementia Discovery Fund is a $100m venture capital fund supported by pharmaceutical companies, governmental organisations and universities globally, specifically focused on providing funding for novel projects resulting in disease-modifying therapies (SV Health Managers LLP n.d.). Other examples of specific funding for dementia research at the national level included Canada (Canadian Institute of Health Research 2017), the UK (Alzheimer's Society, Alzheimer's Research UK and National Institute for Health Research 2017) and Australia (Australian Government 2016). Although these and other new and innovative funding opportunities are promising for dementia research in general, funding technology research specifically will likely continue to be challenging. Much of the development of technologies for dementia exists in the research domain, where funding is provided for specific research projects. Even successful technology research projects can be difficult to translate into products in the hands of users, for example through commercialisation initiatives. The result is that many promising technology projects do not progress beyond the early stages of development, let alone reach real-world trials and commercialisation efforts (Bharucha *et al.* 2009; Czarnuch and Mihailidis 2011). Challenges include limited mechanisms and resources for propelling research outside of a laboratory setting, marginal individual rewards for researchers and intellectual property considerations, among others. For example, who would act as a provider for a technological innovation? Who would pay for manufacturing, distribution and support? Who would assume liability, both during late-phase clinical trials and after? In the current funding model, pharmaceutical companies have often taken on the burden of research, development and translational costs but reap the financial rewards of profitable and successful innovations. Technology development, in most cases, does not follow this model of commercialisation, in many cases because technologies are often focused on dementia as a life issue, rather than a health issue. Examples of this can be clearly seen in earlier chapters in this book. Accordingly, the current and future funding landscape for technology in dementia research is critical to the future of technology innovations in dementia.

Dementia in the future

Consideration of the future of technology innovations in dementia must necessarily include an idea of the future of dementia itself. This includes changes in the underlying population of people who have or will soon develop dementia, as well as our understandings of this population globally. Accordingly, we now briefly consider the changing landscape of dementia demographics globally, as well as our increasing ability to understand dementia around the world.

The changing landscape

Global demographics are changing in an unprecedented way such that the world has an increasing number of older people and a proportionately smaller number of younger people (The World Bank and International Monetary Fund 2016). However, there is considerable heterogeneity demographically across countries, and even regionally within countries, resulting in a diverse set of conditions and needs around the globe (The World Bank and International Monetary Fund 2016). An ageing population has obvious implications for dementia, for example through an increase in both the incidence and prevalence (Alzheimer's Disease International 2015). Additionally, the proportionally fewer young people will be required to support the proportionally larger number of people with dementia in many ways, including financial and social support, as well as serving as informal caregivers. These and other well-documented factors will undoubtedly affect future development of technologies and impact the role that technology will play in dementia care and support.

From a technology innovation perspective, the landscape of an ageing population is also changing in new and unexplored ways that are highly relevant and exciting to the future of dementia innovation, treatment and support. For example, as the first of the baby boomer generation are now over 70 years old, we are likely to see a significant jump in the prevalence of dementia. Research on technology developed to support older adults with dementia has shown mixed results in terms of the applicability and adoption of technologies with older adults with dementia who were in the generation ahead of the boomers. However, the baby boomer generation is much more familiar with technology, including smartphones and computers, as well as the Internet, email and other recent technological advances (e.g. home control systems). This familiarity may lead to better adoption of technologies by older adults with dementia and may allow technology to be used in ways that were not possible with the previous generation. The same can be said for caregivers of people with dementia, who are from the same generation or, in the case of formal caregivers, from a younger generation who have increasingly grown up with digital technologies. Similarly, our newest researchers, clinicians and innovators are emerging from the millennial generation – those reaching adulthood early in the new millennium.

Millennials are not just familiar with technology, but innately speak and understand digital technology and digital language. Millennials, born into digital technology, have been cleverly referred to as 'digital natives', as compared to other generations who have had to learn about technology, acting as 'digital immigrants' (Prensky 2001). This distinction poses an interesting opportunity for the application of technology to dementia in the future. While digital immigrants can still be quite comfortable with technology, their 'accent' is always present to some degree or another. Examples of a technology accent are numerous, such as printing out an email (Prensky 2001). As we move into the future, digital natives will certainly discover new and exciting opportunities for technology in dementia treatment and care. Notably, the concept of digital natives and digital immigrants is largely relevant to the western world, where access to digital technologies is abundant. Indeed, even within more developed western countries, a digital divide can exist between members of different demographics or socioeconomic levels. Globally, a digital divide also exists between countries, easily exemplified when considering developed and developing countries. It is this global digital divide, and the factors that impact and determine access to digital technologies, that we now consider within the context of the future of technology for dementia.

Our global understanding of dementia

Global efforts to fight dementia have helped increase our understandings of dementia on many levels. Perhaps the most sobering statistics have been with respect to the global prevalence (over 46 million people) and cost (818 billion USD annually) of dementia (Alzheimer's Disease International 2016), which indeed have cyclically helped spur interest in global and national action plans. Through early global efforts, we learnt that even a simple understanding of the prevalence of dementia around the world is difficult to obtain because of limited, inconsistent, methodologically variable and even conflicting regional prevalence data (Ferri *et al.* 2005). However, these early efforts resulted in an understanding of the pandemic nature of dementia and began to establish a need for better data and more consistent methodologies in all forms of dementia research and treatment. The result is that we now have a much clearer understanding of the global landscape of dementia, including much more detail about the varied regional impact dementia will have in the future (e.g. Alzheimer's Disease International 2009, 2015). A good example of this is seen through recent estimates suggesting that 58 per cent of people with dementia live in low- or middle-income countries; countries that will also see incidence rates that are approximately double that of high-income countries (Alzheimer's Disease International 2015). From a technology perspective, this is a highly relevant statistic, because the same global estimates also revealed that 94 per cent of people living with dementia in low- or middle-income countries are cared for at home by family members, with little or no access to healthcare. Indeed, many low- and middle-income countries have either limited healthcare delivery infrastructure and services, or limited access to existing healthcare for much of their population. Accordingly, the future of technology innovations is now expanding beyond known markets and applications in high-income countries to potentially help hundreds of other countries around the world in new and exciting ways. These new regions will present new opportunities for development along the design continuum. Innovations may focus on individualised technologies, including user needs assessments through to commercialisation or translation of solutions to the public, such as the use of mobile platforms. Technology development may also focus on institutional and health delivery innovations in regions that do not have a formal healthcare system in place. Certainly, as we continue to learn more about dementia globally, new opportunities will continue to emerge for current and future technology innovations.

Conclusion

The rapid advancements in off-the-shelf consumer technologies in the past 10–15 years have universally increased the pace of innovation. People living with dementia are benefitting from these advances, and as technologies become more intelligent and further able to supplement and enhance human capabilities, we can expect these benefits to continue. In addition, people with dementia will influence these developments as technology co-creators, inventers and champions.

Take-home points

* Technology will play an increasing role in the lives of people with dementia.

* Artificial intelligence offers opportunities for earlier detection and diagnosis of dementia and the implementation of interventions tailored to people's needs.

* Cloud computing and the Internet of Things are creating new opportunities for joined-up systems to empower people to live well with dementia in their own homes.

⋆   People with dementia will play a central role in developing new technologies that meet their needs, priorities and desires.

Acknowledgements

We are grateful to the people living with dementia, their families and caregivers who have shared their experiences and contributed to the development of the ideas expressed in this chapter. We also acknowledge funding for our research from the Canadian Institute of Health Research (CIHR) and AGE-WELL, Canada's ageing and technology network.

References

AAL Association. (n.d.) *About Us.* Retrieved on 23 October 2018 from www.aal-europe.eu/about

Abdollahi, H., Mollahosseini, A., Lane, J. T., & Mahoor, M. H. (2017). A pilot study on using an intelligent life-like robot as a companion for elderly individuals with dementia and depression. In *IEEE-RAS International Conference on Humanoid Robots.* https://doi.org/10.1109/HUMANOIDS.2017.8246925

Alaska Native Tribal Health Consortium (ANTHC). (2016). *About LEO Network: The Eyes, Ears, and Voice of Our Changing Environment.* Retrieved on 28 September 2018 from www.leonetwork.org/en/docs/about/about

Allain, P., Foloppe, D. A., Besnard, J., Yamaguchi, T., *et al.* (2014). Detecting everyday action deficits in Alzheimer's disease using a nonimmersive virtual reality kitchen. *Journal of the International Neuropsychological Society, 20*(5), 468–477.

Allen, F., Cain, R., & Meyer, C. (2018). Seeking relational information sources in the digital age: A study into information source preferences amongst family and friends of those with dementia. *Dementia.* https://doi.org/10.1177/1471301218786568

Alm, N., Astell, A. J., Ellis, M., Dye, R., Gowans, G., & Campbell, J. (2004). A cognitive prosthesis and communication support for people with dementia. *Neuropsychological Rehabilitation, 14*(1), 117–134.

Alm, N., Astell, A. J., Gowans, G., Dye, R., *et al.* (2009). Lessons learned from developing cognitive support for communication, entertainment, and creativity for older people with dementia. In C. Stephanidis (ed.), *Universal Access in Human–Computer Interaction: Addressing Diversity* (Lecture Notes in Computer Science Vol. 5614; pp.195–201). Berlin, Heidelberg: Springer Berlin Heidelberg.

Alm, N., Dye, R., Gowans, G., Campbell, J., Astell, A., & Ellis, M. (2007). A communication support system for older people with dementia. *Computer, 40*(5), 35–41.

Alzheimer Europe. (2010). *The ethical issues linked to the use of assistive technology in dementia care.* Retrieved on 22 October 2018 from www.alzheimer-europe.org/Ethics/Ethical-issues-in-practice/The-ethical-issues-linked-to-the-use-of-assistive-technology-in-dementia-care

Alzheimer Europe. (2014). *Ethical Dilemmas Faced by Carers and People with Dementia.* Luxembourg: Alzheimer Europe. Retrieved on 22 October 2018 from www.alzheimer-europe.org/Ethics/Ethical-issues-in-practice/2014-Ethical-dilemmas-faced-by-carers-and-people-with-dementia

Alzheimer's Association. (2017). *Medications for Memory.* Retrieved on 28 September 2018 from www.alz.org/alzheimers_disease_standard_prescriptions.asp

Alzheimer's Disease International. (2009). *World Alzheimer Report 2009: The Global Prevalence of Dementia.* Retrieved on 28 September 2018 from www.alz.co.uk/research/world-report-2009

Alzheimer's Disease International. (2015). *World Alzheimer Report 2015: The Global Impact of Dementia.* Retrieved on 28 September 2018 from hwww.alz.co.uk/research/world-report-2015

Alzheimer's Disease International. (2016). *World Alzheimer Report 2016: Improving Healthcare for People Living with Dementia.* Retrieved on 28 September 2018 from https://www.alz.co.uk/research/world-report-2016

Alzheimer's Disease International. (n.d.) *Principles of a Dementia Friendly Community.* Retrieved on 28 September 2018 from www.alz.co.uk/dementia-friendly-communities/principles

Alzheimer's Research UK. (2012). *Defeating Dementia: Building Capacity to Capitalise on the UK's Research Strengths.* Retrieved on 28 September 2018 from www.alzheimersresearchuk.org/wp-content/uploads/2015/01/ARUK_Defeating_Dementia_-_Building_capacity_to_capitalise_on_the_UKs_research_strengths.pdf

Alzheimer's Society. (2014). *Alzheimer's Society View On Carer Support: Position Statement.* Retrieved on 28 September 2018 from www.alzheimers.org.uk/info/20091/what_we_think/86/carer_support

Alzheimer's Society. (2015). *Mental Capacity Act 2005.* Retrieved on 28 September 2018 from www.alzheimers.org.uk/download/downloads/id/2646/factsheet_mental_capacity_act_2005.pdf

Alzheimer's Society. (2016a). *Lasting Power of Attorney.* Retrieved on 28 September 2018 from www.alzheimers.org.uk/download/downloads/id/2428/factsheet_lasting_power_of_attorney.pdf

Alzheimer's Society. (2016b). *Carers – Looking After Yourself.* Retrieved on 28 September 2018 from www.alzheimers.org.uk/download/downloads/id/3420/carers_-_looking_after_yourself.pdf

Alzheimer's Society. (2016c). *Coping with Memory Loss.* Factsheet 526LP. Retrieved on 22 October 2018 from www.alzheimers.org.uk/info/20030/staying_independent/30/assistive_technology/6

Alzheimer's Society (2017). *Assistive Technology and Dementia.* Retrieved on 16 January 2019 from https://www.alzheimers.org.uk/get-support/staying-independent/assistive-technology-and-dementia#content-start

Alzheimer's Society, Alzheimer's Research UK & National Institute for Health Research. (2017). *Funding Opportunities: Dementia research funding portal.* Retrieved on 28 September 2018 from http://dementiaresearchfunding.org.uk/about-us

Amazon Web Services. (2006). *Announcing Amazon Elastic Compute Cloud (Amazon EC2) – beta.* Retrieved on 7 October 2017 from https://aws.amazon.com/about-aws/whats-new/2006/08/24/announcing-amazon-elastic-compute-cloud-amazon-ec2---beta/

American Psychiatric Association. (2013). *Diagnostic and Statistical Manual of Mental Disorders.* Arlington, TX: American Psychiatric Association.

Amiribesheli, M. & Bouchachia, A. (2017). A tailored smart home for dementia care. *Journal of Ambient Intelligence and Humanized Computing.* https://doi.org/org/10.1007/s1265

Arntzen, C., Holthe, T., & Jentoft, R. (2016). Tracing the successful incorporation of assistive technology into everyday life for younger people with dementia and family carers. *Dementia, 15*(4), 646–662.

Astell, A. J. (2006). Technology and personhood in dementia care. *Quality in Ageing and Older Adults, 7*(1), 15–25.

Astell, A. J., Alm, N., Dye, R., Gowans, G., Vaughan, P., & Ellis, M. (2014a). Digital Video Games for Older Adults with Cognitive Impairment. In K. Miesenberger, D. Fels, D. Archambault, P. Peňáz, & W. Zagler (eds), *Computers Helping People with Special Needs* (Lecture Notes in Computer Science Vol. 8547; pp.264–271). Cham: Springer International.

Astell, A. J., Alm, N., Gowans, G., Ellis, M. P., Dye, R., & Campbell, J. (2008). CIRCA: A Communication Prosthesis for Dementia. In A. Mihailidis, J. Boger, H. Kautz, & L. Normie (eds), *Technology and Aging* (Assistive Technology Research Series Vol. 21; pp.67–76). Amsterdam: IOS Press.

Astell, A. J., Alm, N., Gowans, G., Ellis, M., Dye, R., & Vaughan, P. (2009). Involving older people with dementia and their carers in designing computer based support systems: Some methodological considerations. *Universal Access in the Information Society, 8*, 49–58.

Astell, A. J., Czarnuch, S., & Dove, E. (2018a). System development guidelines from a review of motion-based technology for people with dementia or MCI. *Frontiers in Psychiatry, 9.* https://doi.org/10.3389/fpsyt.2018.00189

Astell, A. J., Ellis, M. P., Bernardi, L., Alm, N., *et al.* (2010). Using a touch screen computer to support relationships between people with dementia and caregivers. *Interacting with Computers, 22*(4), 267–275.

Astell, A. J., Joddrell, P., Groenewoud, H., de Lange, J., *et al.* (2016). Does familiarity affect the enjoyment of touchscreen games for people with dementia? *International Journal of Medical Informatics, 91,* e1–e8.

Astell, A. J., Malone, B., Williams, G., Hwang, F., & Ellis, M. P. (2014b). Leveraging everyday technology for people living with dementia: A case study. *Journal of Assistive Technologies, 8*(4), 164–176.

Astell, A. J., Smith, S. K., Potter, S., & Preston-Jones, E. (2018b). Computer interactive reminiscence and conversation aid groups: Delivering cognitive stimulation with technology. *Alzheimer's & Dementia: Translational Research & Clinical Interventions, 4,* 481–487.

AT Dementia. (2017). *The ethical use of assistive technology.* Retrieved on 22 October 2018 from www.atdementia.org.uk/editorial.asp?page_id=47

Australian Government. (2016). *Boosting Dementia Research Initiative.* Retrieved on 28 September 2018 from www.nhmrc.gov.au/research/boosting-dementia-research-initiative

Bail, K. D. (2003). Electronic tagging of people with dementia: Devices may be preferable to locked doors. *British Medical Journal, 326*(7383), 281.

Baldwin, C. (2005). Technology dementia and ethics: Rethinking the issues. *Disability Studies Quarterly, 25*(3). Retrieved on 28 September 2018 from www.dsq-sds.org/article/view/583/760

Balebako, R., Marsh, A., Lin, J., Hong, J., & Cranor, L. F. (2014). *The Privacy and Security Behaviors of Smartphone App Developers.* Workshop on Usable Security. Retrieved on 22 October 2018 from http://lorrie.cranor.org/pubs/usec14-app-developers.pdf

Bartlett, R., & O'Connor, D. (2007). From personhood to citizenship: Broadening the lens for dementia practice and research. *Journal of Aging Studies, 21*(2), 107–118.

Bartlett, R., & O'Connor, D. (2010). *Broadening the Dementia Debate: Towards Social Citizenship.* Bristol: Policy Press.

Batsch, N. L., & Mittelman, M. S. (2012). *World Alzheimer Report 2012: Overcoming the Stigma of Dementia.* London: Alzheimer's Disease International.

Beauchamp, J., & Childress, J. (2009). *Principles of Biomedical Ethics,* 6th edition. New York, NY: Oxford University Press.

Beeharee, A., & Steed, A. (2006). A natural wayfinding exploiting photos in pedestrian navigation systems. In *MobileHCI '06 Proceedings of the 8th Conference on Human–Computer Interaction with Mobile Devices and Services.* https://doi.org/10.1145/1152215.1152233

Benbow, S. M., & Jolley, D. (2012). Dementia: Stigma and its effects. *Neurodegenerative Disease Management, 2*(2012), 165–172.

Bewernitz, M. W., Mann, W. C., Dasler, P., & Belchior, P. (2009). Feasibility of machine-based prompting to assist persons with dementia. *Assistive Technology: The Official Journal of RESNA, 21,* 196–207.

Bhagyashree, S. I. R., Nagaraj, K., Prince, M., Fall, C. H. D., & Krishna, M. (2017). Diagnosis of dementia by machine learning methods in epidemiological studies: A pilot exploratory study from South India. *Social Psychiatry and Psychiatric Epidemiology,* 1–10. doi:10.1007/s00127-017-1410-0

Bharucha, A. J., Anand, V., Forlizzi, J., Dew, M. A., *et al.* (2009). Intelligent assistive technology applications to dementia care: Current capabilities, limitations, and future challenges. *American Journal of Geriatric Psychiatry, 17*(2), 88–104.

Bødker, S. (1993). The AT Project: Practical Research in Cooperative Design. *DAIMI Report Series, 22*(454). https://doi.org/10.7146/dpb.v22i454.6772.

Boman, I-L., Lundberg, S., Starkhammar, S., & Nygård, L. (2014a). Exploring the usability of a videophone mock-up for people with dementia and their significant others. *BMC Geriatrics, 14,* 49.

Boman, I.-L., Nygård, L., and Rosenberg, L. (2014b). Users' and professionals' contributions in the process of designing an easy-to-use videophone for people with dementia. *Disability and Rehabilitation: Assistive Technology 9,* 2, 164–172.

Bonney, R., Cooper, C. B., Dickinson, J., Kelling, S., *et al.* (2009). Citizen science: A developing tool for expanding science knowledge and scientific literacy. *BioScience, 59*(11), 977–984.

Boots, L. M. M., de Vugt, M. E., van Knippenberg, R. J. M., Kempen, G. I. J. M., & Verhey, F. R. J. (2014). A systematic review of Internet-based supportive interventions for caregivers of patients with dementia. *International Journal of Geriatric Psychiatry, 29*(4), 331–344.

Bovbel, P. & Nejat, G. (2014). Casper: An assistive kitchen robot to promote aging in place. *Journal of medical devices, 8*(3), 030945.

Bowes, A. & McColgan, G. (2006). *Smart Technology and Community Care for Older People: Innovation in West Lothian, Scotland.* Edinburgh: Age Concern Scotland.

Bowes, A. & McColgan, G. (2013). Telecare for older people: Promoting independence, participation and identity. *Research on Ageing, 35*(1), 32–49.

Branco, R. M., Quental, J., & Ribeiro, Ó. (2015). Getting closer, empathising and understanding: Setting the stage for a codesign project with people with dementia. *Interaction Design and Architecture, 26,* 114–131.

Brankaert, R. (2016). *Design for dementia: A design-driven living lab approach to involve people living with dementia and their context.* PhD thesis, University of Technology Eindhoven, Eindhoven. https://doi.org/978-90-386-4030-3

Brankaert, R. & den Ouden, E. (2017). The design-driven living lab: A new approach to exploring solutions to complex societal challenges. *Technology Innovation Management Review.* Retrieved on 4 October 2018 from https://timreview.ca/article/1049

Brankaert, R., den Ouden, E., & Brombacher, A. (2015). Innovate dementia: The development of a living lab protocol to evaluate interventions in context. *Info.* https://doi.org/10.1108/info-01-2015-0010

Brennan, P. F., Moore, S. M., & Smyth, K. A. (1991). ComputerLink: Electronic support for the home caregiver. *Annals of Advanced Nursing Science, 13*(4), 14–27.

Brittain, K., Corner, L., Robinson, L., & Bond, J. (2010). Ageing in place and technologies of place: The lived experience of people with dementia in changing social, physical and technological environments. *Sociology of Health and Illness, 32*(2), 272–287.

Brorsson, A., Öhman, A., Lundberg, S., & Nygård, L. (2011). Accessibility in public space as perceived by people with Alzheimer's disease. *Dementia, 10*(4), 587–602.

Buffel, T., Phillipson, C., & Scharf, T. (2012). Ageing in urban environments: Developing 'age-friendly' cities. *Critical Social Policy, 32*(4), 597–617.

Burrow, S. & Brooks, D. (2012). ATDementia: An information resource on assistive technologies that help support the independence of people with dementia. *Dementia, 11*(4), 553–557.

Cabral, C., Morgado, P. M., Campos Costa, D., & Silveira, M. (2015). Predicting conversion from MCI to AD with FDG-PET brain images at different prodromal stages. *Computers in Biology and Medicine, 58,* 101–109.

Caffò, A. O., Hoogeveen, F., Groenendaal, M., Perilli, A. V., *et al.* (2014). Intervention strategies for spatial orientation disorders in dementia: A selective review. *Developmental Neurorehabilitation, 17*(3), 200–209.

Camic, P. M., Baker, E. L., & Tischler, V. (2016). Theorizing how art gallery interventions impact people with dementia and their caregivers. *Gerontologist, 56*(6), 1033–1041.

Canadian Institute of Health Research. (2017). *CIHR Dementia Research Strategy.* Retrieved on 28 September 2018 from www.cihr-irsc.gc.ca/e/43629.html

Cannon, J. C. (2005). *Privacy: What Developers and IT Professionals Should Know.* Harlow: Addison-Wesley.

Capus, J. (2005). The Kingston Dementia Café: The benefits of establishing an Alzheimer café for carers and people with dementia. *Dementia, 4*(4), 588–591.

Care Quality Commission. (2015). *Thinking About Using a Hidden Camera or Other Equipment to Monitor Someone's Care?* Newcastle upon Tyne: Care Quality Commission. Retrieved on 28 September 2018 from www.cqc.org.uk/sites/default/files/20150212_public_surveillance_leaflet_final.pdf

Carers Trust. (2015). *Caring About Older Carers: Providing Support for People Caring Later in Life.* London: Carers Trust. Retrieved on 23 October 2018 from https://professionals.carers.org/sites/default/files/caring_about_older_carers.pdf

Carers UK. (2012). *Future Care: Care and Technology for the 21st Century.* London: Carers Trust. Retrieved on 28 September 2018 from www.carersuk.org/for-professionals/policy/policy-library/future-care-care-and-technology-in-the-21st-century

Cavoukian, A. (2011). *The 7 Foundational Principles: Implementation and Mapping of Fair Information Practices.* Retrieved on 22 October 2018 from http://www.ontla.on.ca/library/repository/mon/24005/301946.pdf

Cavoukian, A. (2012). Privacy by Design: Origins, Meaning, and Prospects for Assuring Privacy and Trust in the Information Era. In G. Yee (ed.), *Privacy Protection Measures and Technologies in Business Organizations: Aspects and Standards* (pp.170–208). Hershey, PA: IGI Global.

Chakrabarti, S., Ester, M., Fayyad, U., Gehrke, J., *et al.* (2006). *Data Mining Curriculum: A Proposal (Version 1.0).* Retrieved on 29 September 2018 from www.kdd.org/exploration_files/CURMay06.pdf

Chalghoumi, H., Cobigo, V., Dignard, C., Gauthier-Beaupré, A., *et al.* (2017). Information privacy for technology users with intellectual and developmental disabilities: Why does it matter? *Ethics and Behavior.* doi: 10.1080/10508422.2017.1393340

Chen, P. H., Yang, M. H., & Lee, D. D. (2016). *Data Mining the Co-Morbid Associations Between Dementia and Various Kinds of Illnesses Using a Medicine Database.* Paper presented at the International Conference on Green Technology and Sustainable Development (GTSD), Kaohsiung, Taiwan, 24–25 November.

Cheng, B., Liu, M., Zhang, D., Munsell, B. C., & Shen, D. (2015). Domain transfer learning for MCI conversion prediction. *IEEE Transactions on Biomedical Engineering, 62*(7), 1805–1817.

Clark, J. & McGee-Lennon, M. (2011). A stakeholder-centred exploration of the current barriers to the uptake of home care technology in the UK. *Journal of Assistive Technologies, 5*(1), 12–25.

Clarke, A., Hanson, E. J., & Ross, H. (2003). Seeing the person behind the patient: Enhancing the care of older people using a biographical approach. *Journal of Clinical Nursing, 12*(5), 697–706.

Clasper, K. (2018). *Living Well with Lewy Body Dementia and Comorbidities.* Retrieved on 28 September 2018 from http://ken-kenc2.blogspot.co.uk

Coradeschi, S., Cesta, A., Cortellessa, G., Coraci, L., *et al.* (2013). GiraffPlus: Combining social interaction and long term monitoring for promoting independent living. In *2013 6th International Conference on Human System Interactions, HSI 2013,* Rzeszow, Poland 6–8 June (pp.578–585).

Coughlin, J. (2015). When robots begin to care. *Huffpost,* 9 May. Retrieved on 22 October 2018 from www.huffingtonpost.com/joseph-f-coughlin/when-robots-begin-to-care_b_6826022.html

Cousins, S. (2017). New tool to improve dementia design. *Royal Institute of British Architects Journal.* Retrieved on 29 September 2018 from www.ribaj.com/products/living-with-dementia

Crampton, J., & Eley, R. (2013). Dementia-friendly communities: What the project 'Creating a dementia-friendly York' can tell us. *Working with Older People, 17*(2), 49–57.

Cristancho-Lacroix, V., Moulin, F., Wrobel, J., Batrancourt, B., *et al.* (2014). A web-based program for informal caregivers of persons with Alzheimer's disease: An iterative user-centered design. *JMIR Research Protocols, 3*(3), e46.

Critten, V. & Kucirkova, N. (2017). 'It brings it all back, all those good times; it makes me go close to tears': Creating digital personalised stories with people who have dementia. *Dementia.* https://doi.org/10.1177/1471301217691162

Ctrl Group. (2017). *Dementia Citizens Beta: Creating a citizen science platform for people with dementia and their carers.* Retrieved on 28 September 2018 from www.ctrl-group.com/projects/dementia-citizens

Cui, Y., Liu, B., Luo, S., Zhen, X., *et al.* (2011). Identification of conversion from mild cognitive impairment to Alzheimer's disease using multivariate predictors. *PloS One, 6*(7), e21896.

Cushman, L. A., Stein, K., & Duffy, C. J. (2008). Detecting navigational deficits in cognitive aging and Alzheimer disease using virtual reality. *Neurology, 71*(12), 888–895.

Czarnuch, S., Cohen, S., Parameswaran, V., & Mihailidis, A. (2013). A real-world deployment of the COACH prompting system. *Journal of Ambient Intelligence and Smart Environments, Thematic Issue on Designing and Deploying Intelligent Environments, 5*(4), 463–478.

Czarnuch, S. & Mihailidis, A. (2011). The design of intelligent in-home assistive technologies: Assessing the needs of older adults with dementia and their caregivers. *Gerontechnology, 10*(3), 165–178.

Czarnuch, S., Ricciardelli, R., & Mihailidis, A. (2016). Predicting the role of assistive technologies in the lives of people with dementia using objective care recipient factors. *BMC Geriatrics, 16*(1), 1–11.

Dabelko-Schoeny, H., Phillips, G., Darrough, E., DeAnna, S., *et al.* (2014). Equine-assisted intervention for people with dementia. *Anthrozoos, 27*(1), 141–155.

Daily Caring. (2017). *Amazon Echo for Dementia: Technology for seniors.* Retrieved on 29 September 2018 from http://dailycaring.com/amazon-echo-for-dementia-technology-for-seniors

Dallora, A. L., Eivazzadeh, S., Mendes, E., Berglund, J., & Anderberg, P. (2017). Machine learning and microsimulation techniques on the prognosis of dementia: A systematic literature review. *PloS One, 12*(6), e0179804.

Deetjen, U., Meyer, E. T., & Schroeder, R. (2015). *Big Data for Advancing Dementia Research: An Evaluation of Data Sharing Practices in Research on Age-related Neurodegenerative Diseases.* OECD Digital Economy Papers, No. 246. Paris: OECD Publishing.

Del Campo, A., Gambi, E., Montanini, L., Perla, D., Raffaeli, L., & Spinsante, S. (2016). *MQTT in AAL Systems for Home Monitoring of People with Dementia.* Paper presented at the IEEE Annual International Symposium on Personal, Indoor, and Mobile Radio Communications (PIMRC), Valencia, Spain, 4–8 September.

Deloitte. (2017). *State of the Smart: Consumer and Business Usage Patterns. Global Mobile Consumer Survey 2017: UK Cut.* Retrieved on 23 October 2018 at www.deloitte.co.uk/mobileuk2017/assets/img/download/global-mobile-consumer-survey-2017_uk-cut.pdf?_ga=2.10701428.1165717553.1539705271-503998821.1539705271

Depaoli, P. (2016). Organizing e-Services Co-production in Multiple Contexts: Implications for Designers and Policymakers. In F. D'Ascenzo, M. Magni, A. Lazazzara, & S. Za (eds), *Blurring the Boundaries Through Digital Innovation* (Lecture Notes in Information Systems and Organisation Vol. 19; pp. 231–245). Cham: Springer.

Department of Health. (2005). *Building Telecare in England.* London: Department of Health.

Department of Health. (2015). *Prime Minister's Challenge on Dementia 2020.* London: Department of Health.

Department of Health and Social Care. (2012). *One million 'Dementia Friends' will help make life better for people with dementia.* Retrieved on 29 September 2018 from www.gov.uk/government/news/one-million-dementia-friends-will-help-make-life-better-for-people-with-dementia de Vugt, M. & Dröes, R.-M. (2017). Social health in dementia. Towards a positive dementia discourse. *Aging and Mental Health, 21*(1), 1–3.

Dewey, J. (1981). *The Later Works, 1925–1953*, J. A. Boydston (ed.). Carbondale, IL: Southern Illinois University Press.

Dierkx, R., Heshof, N., & Remmerswaal, M. (2017). *Bewegingsvrijheid en mobiliteit Maximaliseren en optimaliseren bij bewoners met dementie.* Retrieved on 26 March 2018, from www. verensotijdschrift.nl/om2017/november-2017/wetenschap/bewegingsvrijheid-en-mobiliteit/#.WhK3N0ribcs

Di Lorito, C., Birt, L., Poland, F., Csipke, E., *et al.* (2017). A synthesis of the evidence on peer research with potentially vulnerable adults: How this relates to dementia. *International Journal of Geriatric Psychiatry, 32*(1), 58–67.

Dimitrioglou, N., Kardaras, D., & Barbounaki, S. (2017). Multicriteria Evaluation of the Internet of Things Potential in Health Care: The Case of Dementia Care. Paper presented at the IEEE Conference on Business Informatics (CBI), Thessaloniki, Greece, 24–27 July.

Dixon, J. (2016). *Technology Integrated Health Management: Insight into the Needs of Citizens with Dementia, Those Who Care for Them and Clinicians.* Leatherhead: Surrey and Borders Partnership NHS Foundation Trust. Retrieved on 28 March 2018 from www.sabp.nhs. uk/application/files/9615/1603/2365/TIHM_Insights_Report.pdf

Doubal, F. N., Ali, M., Batty, G. D., Charidimou, A., *et al.* (2017). Big data and data repurposing: Using existing data to answer new questions in vascular dementia research. *BMC Neurology, 17*(72). doi:10.1186/s12883-017-0841-2

Dove, E. & Astell, A. J. (2017a). Dementia: Kinecting through group digital games. *Journal of Dementia Care, 26*(1), 18–19.

Dove, E. & Astell, A. J. (2017b). The Kinect Project: Group motion-based gaming for people living with dementia. *Dementia, 0*(0), 1–17. doi: 10.1177/1471301217743575

Dove, E. & Astell, A. J. (2017c). The use of motion-based technology for people living with dementia or mild cognitive impairment: A literature review. *Journal of Medical Internet Research, 19*(1), e3.

Dove, E. Cotnam, K., & Astell, A. J. (2017). Exploring the use of group digital activities for people living with dementia. *Innovation in Aging, 1*(suppl. 1). https://doi.org/10.1093/geroni/igx004.1726

Downes, J. J., Roberts, A. C., Sahakian, B. J., Evenden, J. L., Morris, R. G., & Robbins, T. W. (1989). Impaired extra-dimensional shift performance in medicated and unmedicated Parkinson's disease: Evidence for a specific attentional dysfunction. *Neuropsychologia, 27*(11–12), 1329–1343.

Eichler, T., Thyrian, J. R., Hertel, J., Richter, S., *et al.* (2016). Unmet needs of commuity-dwelling primary care patients with dementia in Germany: Prevalence and correlates. *Journal of Alzheimer's Disease, 51*(3), 847–855.

Ekström, A., Ferm, U., & Samuelsson, C. (2015). Digital communication support and Alzheimer's disease. *Dementia, 16*(6), 711–731.

Emmons, R., & Mishra, A. (2011). Why Gratitude Enhances Wellbeing: What We Know, What We Need to Know. In K. M. Sheldon, T. B. Kashdan and M. F. Steger, (eds), *Designing Positive Psychology: Taking Stock and Moving Forward* (pp.228–247). Oxford: Oxford University Press.

Enshaeifar, S., Barnaghi, P., Skillman, S., Markides, A., *et al.* (2018). Internet of Things for dementia care. *IEEE Internet Computing, 22*(1), 8–17.

Essén, A. (2008). The two facets of electronic care surveillance: An exploration of the views of older people who live with monitoring devices. *Social Science and Medicine, 67*(1), 128–136.

Evans, S. C., Garabedien, S., & Bray, J. (2017). 'Now he sings'. The My Musical Memories Reminiscence Programmes: Personalised interactive reminiscence sessions for people living with dementia. *Dementia.* https://doi.org/10.1177/1471301217710531

Fels, D. I. & Astell, A. J. (2011). Storytelling as a model of conversation for people with dementia and caregivers. *American Journal of Alzheimer's Disease and Other Dementias, 26*(7), 535–541.

Fereshtehnejad, S.-M., Damangir, S., Cermakova, P., Aarsland, D., Eriksdotter, M., & Religa, D. (2014). Comorbidity profile in dementia with Lewy bodies versus Alzheimer's disease: A linkage study between the Swedish Dementia Registry and the Swedish National Patient Registry. *Alzheimer's Research and Therapy, 6*(5), 65.

Ferri, C. P., Prince, M., Brayne, C., Brodaty, H., *et al.* (2005). Global prevalence of dementia: A Delphi consensus study. *Lancet, 366*(9503), 2112–2117.

Fisk, M. (2015). Surveillance technologies in care homes: Seven principles for their use. *Working with Older People, 19*(2), 51–59.

Forestry Commission. (2011). *Action Plan for Tree Health and Plant Biosecurity.* Retrieved on 28 September 2018 from www.forestry.gov.uk/pdf/Action-Plan-Tree-health-and-plant-biosecurity.pdf/$FILE/Action-Plan-Tree-health-and-plant-biosecurity.pdf

Foundation for Assistive Technology, Innovations in Dementia and Trent DSDC. (2011). *Getting Equipped to Tackle Forgetfulness: Top Tips for Family and Friends.* London: Foundation for Assistive Technology. Retrieved on 28 September 2018 from www.thinklocalactpersonal.org.uk/_assets/Resources/Personalisation/Carers/Innovationfund/Getting_equipped_to_tackle_forgetfulness.pdf

Fraser, K. C., Meltzer, J. A., & Rudzicz, F. (2016). Linguistic features identify Alzheimer's disease in narrative speech. *Journal of Alzheimer's Disease, 49*(2), 407–422.

Friedman, B., Kahn Jr, P. H., Borning, A., & Huldtgren, A. (2013). Value Sensitive Design and Information Systems. In N. Doorne, D. Schuurbiers, I. van de Poel & E. Gorman (eds), *Early Engagement and New Technologies: Opening up the Laboratory* (pp.55–95). Dordretch: Springer.

Galvin, J. E., Meuser, T. M., Coats, M. A., Bakal, D. A., & Morris, J. C. (2009). The 'portable' CDR: Translating the Clinical Dementia Rating Interview into a PDA format. *Alzheimer Disease and Associated Disorders, 23*(1), 44–49.

García-Betances, R. I., Arredondo Waldmeyer, M. T., Fico, G., & Cabrera-Umpiérrez, M. F. (2015). A succinct overview of virtual reality technology use in Alzheimer's disease. *Frontiers in Aging Neuroscience, 7,* 80.

Garrido, S., Dunne, L., Chang, E., Perz, J., Stevens, C. J., & Haertsch, M. (2017). The use of music playlists for people with dementia: A critical synthesis. *Journal of Alzheimer's Disease, 60*(3), 1129–1142.

Gastmans, C. (2013). Dignity-enhancing nursing care: A foundational ethical framework. *Nursing Ethics, 2*(42), 142–149.

Gibson, G., Dickinson, C., Brittain, K., & Robinson, L. (2015). The everyday use of assistive technology by people with dementia and their family carers: A qualitative study. *BMC Geriatrics, 15*(89). https://doi.org/10.1186/s12877-015-0091-3

Gibson, G., Newton, L., Pritchard, G., Finch, T., Brittain, K., & Robinson, L. (2016). The provision of assistive technology products and services for people with dementia in the United Kingdom. *Dementia, 15*(4), 681–701.

Godwin, B. (2012). The ethical evaluation of assistive technology for practitioners: A checklist arising from a participatory study with people with dementia, family and professionals. *Journal of Assistive Technologies, 6*(2), 123–135.

Goodman, J., Brewster, S. A., & Gray, P. (2005). How can we best use landmarks to support older people in navigation? *Journal of Behaviour and Information Technology, 24,* 3–20.

Google. (2013). Google Compute Engine is now generally available with expanded OS support, transparent maintenance, and lower prices. *Google Cloud Platform Blog.* Retrieved on 7 October 2018 from https://cloudplatform.googleblog.com/2013/12/google-compute-engine-is-now-generally-available.html

Grand, J. H. G., Caspar, S., & MacDonald, S. W. S. (2011). Clinical features and multidisciplinary approaches to dementia care. *Journal of Multidisciplinary Healthcare, 4,* 125–147.

Greenhalgh, T. (2012). Whole system demonstrator trial: Policy, politics and publication ethics. *BMJ, 345,* 7869.

Greenhalgh, T., Procter, R., Wherton, J., Sugarhood, P., Hinder, S., & Rouncefield, M. (2015). What is quality in assisted living technology? The ARCHIE framework for effective telehealth and telecare services, *BMC Medicine*, *13*, 91.

Greenhalgh, T., Procter, R., Wherton, J., Sugarhood, P., & Shaw, S. (2012). The organising vision for telehealth and telecare: Discourse analysis. *BMJ Open*, *2*, e001574.

Greenhalgh, T., Wherton, J., Papoutsi, C., Lynch, J., *et al.* (2017). Beyond adoption: A new framework for theorizing and evaluating nonadoption, abandonment and challenges to the scale-up, spread and sustainability of health and care technologies. *Journal of Medical Informatics Research*, *19*(11), e367.

Greenhalgh, T., Wherton, J., Sugarhood, P., Hinder, S., & Procter, R. (2013). What matters to older people with assisted living needs? A phenomenological analysis of the use and non-use of telehealth and telecare. *Social Science and Medicine*, *93*, 86–94.

Grossman, M. R., Zak, D. K., & Zelinski, E. M. (2018). Mobile apps for caregivers of older adults: Quantitative content analysis. *JMIR mHealth and uHealth*, *6*(7), e162.

Hagethorn, F. N., Kröse, B. J. A., De Greef, P., & Helmer, M. E. (2008). Creating Design Guidelines for a Navigational Aid for Mild Demented Pedestrians. In E. Aarts, J. L. Crowley, B. de Ruyter, H. Gerhäuser, A. Pflaum, J. Schmidt, & R. Wichert (eds), *Ambient Intelligence: European Conference, AmI 2008* (Lecture Notes in Computer Science Vol 5355; pp. 276–289). Berlin, Heidelberg: Springer Berlin Heidelberg.

HammondCare. (2017). *Annual Report 2017*. Sydney, Australia: HammondCare.

Hattink, B., Meiland, F., van der Roest, H., Kevern, P., *et al.* (2015). Web-based STAR e-learning course increases empathy and understanding in dementia caregivers: Results from a randomized controlled trial in the Netherlands and the United Kingdom. *Journal of Medical Internet Research*, *17*(10), e241.

Hedman, A., Lindqvist, E., & Nygård, L. (2016). How older adults with mild cognitive impairment relate to technology as part of present and future everyday life: A qualitative study. *BMC Geriatrics*, *16*(1), 73.

Hemment, D., Ellis, R., & Wynne, B. (2011). Participatory mass observation and citizen science. *Leonardo*, *44*(1), 62–63.

Henderson, C., Knapp, M., Fernandez, J., Beecham, J., *et al.* (2014). Cost-effectiveness of telecare for people with social care needs: The Whole Systems Demonstrator cluster randomised trial. *Age and Ageing*, *43*(6), 794–800.

Hendriks, N., Huybrechts, L., Wilkinson, A., & Slegers, K. (2014). Challenges in doing participatory design with people with dementia. In *Proceedings of the 13th Participatory Design Conference: Short Papers, Industry Cases, Workshop Descriptions, Doctoral Consortium papers, and Keynote Abstracts. PDC 2014*, Vol. 2 (pp.33–36). New York: ACM.

Hernandez, A., Astell, A., & Theiventhiran, D. (2017). Introducing touch screen applications to people with advanced dementia through staff–client co-play. *Innovation in Aging*, *1*(1), 482–483.

Hesook, S. E. (2017). Assistive Technology for People with Dementia: Ethical Considerations. In I. Kollak (ed.), *Safe at Home with Assistive Technology* (pp.173–191). Berlin: Springer.

Hettinga, M., De Boer, J., Goldberg, E., & Moelaert, F. (2009). Navigation for people with mild dementia. *Studies in Health Technology and Informatics*, *150*, 428–432.

Hobday, J. V., Savik, K., Smith, S., & Gaugler, J. E. (2010). Feasibility of Internet training for care staff of residents with dementia: The CARES program. *Journal of Gerontological Nursing*, *36*(4), 13–21.

Hofmann, M., Hock, C., Kühler, A., & Müller-Spahn, F. (1996). Interactive computer-based cognitive training in patients with Alzheimer's disease. *Journal of Psychiatric Research*, *30*(6), 493–501.

Hofmann-Apitius, M. (2015). Is dementia research ready for big data approaches? *BMC Medicine*, *13*(1), 145.

Hofstadter, D. R. (1979). *Gödel, Escher, Bach: An Eternal Golden Braid*. London: Penguin.

Holbø, K., Bøthun, S., & Dahl, Y. (2013). Safe Walking Technology for People with Dementia: What Do They Want? In *Proceedings of the 15th International ACM SIGACCESS Conference on Computers and Accessibility.* https://doi.org/10.1145/2513383.2513434

Hughes, C. P., Berg, L., Danziger, W. L., Coben, L. A., & Martin, R. L. (1982). A new clinical scale for the staging of dementia. *British Journal of Psychiatry, 140,* 566–572.

Hughes, J. C. & Baldwin, C. (2006). *Ethical Issues in Dementia Care.* London: Jessica Kingsley Publishers.

Hughes, J. C. & Louw, S. J. (2002). Electronic tagging of people with dementia who wander. *BMJ (Clinical Research edn), 325,* 847–848.

Hussey, J. (2016). Younger people: An innovative partnership. *Journal of Dementia Care, 24*(6), 20–22.

Ienca, M., Fabrice, J., Elger, B., Caon, M., *et al.* (2017). Intelligent assistive technology for Alzheimer's disease and other dementias: A systematic review. *Journal of Alzheimer's Disease, 56*(4), 1301–1340.

Ienca, M., Wangmo, T., Jotterand, F., Kressig, R. W., & Elger, B. (2018). Ethical design of intelligent assistive technologies for dementia: A descriptive review. *Science and Engineering Ethics, 24*(4), 1035–1055.

Imbeault, H., Bier, N., Pigot, H., Gagnon, L., Marcotte, N., Fulop, T., & Giroux, S. (2014). Electronic organiser and Alzheimer's disease: Fact or fiction? *Neuropsychological Rehabilitation, 24*(1), 71–100.

INDEX. (2011, 9 November). Nursebot: Personal mobile robotic assistants for the elderly. Retrieved on 29 September 2018 from https://designtoimprovelife.dk/nursebot-personal-mobile-robotic-assistants-for-the-elderly

International Organization for Standardization. (2018). *ISO 9241-11:2018.* Retrieved on 15 October 2018 from www.iso.org/obp/ui/#iso:std:iso:9241:-11:ed-2:v1:en

Irwin, A. (1995). *Citizen Science: A Study of People, Expertise and Sustainable Development.* London: Routledge.

Jacobsen, J. H., Stelzer, J., Fritz, T. H., Chételat, G., La Joie, R., & Turner, R. (2015). Why musical memory can be preserved in advanced Alzheimer's disease. *Brain, 138*(March), 2438–2450.

Joddrell, P. (2017). *Investigating the potential of touchscreen technology to create opportunities for independent activity with people living with dementia.* PhD thesis, University of Sheffield, Faculty of Medicine, Dentistry and Health, School of Health and Related Research, Sheffield.

Joddrell, P. & Astell, A. J. (2016). Studies involving people with dementia and touchscreen technology: A literature review. *JMIR Rehabilitation and Assistive Technologies, 3*(2), e10.

Joddrell, P., Hernandez, A., & Astell, A. J. (2016). Identifying existing, accessible touchscreen games for people living with dementia. In K. Miesenberger, C. Buhler, & P. Penaz (eds), *Computers Helping People with Special Needs* (Lecture Notes in Computer Science Vol. 9758; pp.509–514). Berlin: Springer International Publishing.

Keady, J., Hyden, L., Johnson, A. & and Swarbrick, C. (eds) (2018). *Social Research Methods in Dementia Studies: Including and Innovation.* Abingdon: Routledge.

Kellet, U., Moyle, W., McAllister, M., King, C., & Gallagher, F. (2010). Life stories and biography: A means of connecting family and staff for people with dementia. *Journal of Clinical Nursing, 19*(11–12), 1707–1715.

Kenner, A. (2008). Securing the elderly body: Dementia, surveillance and the politics of 'aging in place'. *Surveillance and Society, 5*(3), 252–269.

Kessels, R., de Werd, M. M., Boelen, D., & Olde Rikkert, M. (2013). Errorless learning of everyday tasks in people with dementia. *Clinical Interventions in Aging, 8,* 1177–1190.

Killin, L., Russ, T., Surdhar, S., Yoon, Y., *et al.* (2018). The Digital Support Platform: Investigating the feasibility of an internet-based, post diagnostic support platform for families living with dementia. *BMJ Open, 8*(4), e020281.

König, A., Crispim-Junior, C. F., Covella, A. G. U., Bremond, F., *et al.* (2015a). Ecological assessment of autonomy in instrumental activities of daily living in dementia patients by the means of an automatic video monitoring system. *Frontiers in Aging Neuroscience, 7*(June). https://doi.org/10.3389/fnagi.2015.00098

König, A., Satt, A., Sorin, A., Hoory, R., *et al.* (2015b). Automatic speech analysis for the assessment of patients with predementia and Alzheimer's disease. *Alzheimer's and Dementia: Diagnosis, Assessment and Disease Monitoring, 1*(1), 112–124.

Kontos, P. C. (2005). Embodied selfhood in Alzheimer's disease: Rethinking person-centred care. *Dementia, 4*(4), 553–570.

Korebrits, G., Gajjarr, A., & Palmer, S. (2017). The joy and freedom of dance. *Australian Journal of Dementia Care,* 4 June. Retrieved on 23 October 2017 from http://journalofdementiacare.com/the-joy-and-freedom-of-dance

Kottorp, A. & Nygård, L. (2011). Development of a short form assessment for everyday technology used with older adults with MCI or Alzheimer's disease. *Expert Review of Neurotherapeutics, 11*(5), 647–655.

Kristoffersson, A., Coradeschi, S., & Loutfi, A. (2013). A review of mobile robotic telepresence. *Advances in Human-Computer Interaction.* https://doi.org/10.1155/2013/902316

Krogstie, J. (2012). Bridging Research and Innovation by Applying Living Labs for Design Science Research. In *Nordic Contributions in IS Research* (Lecture Notes in Business Information Processing Vol. 124; pp.161–176). Berlin, Heidelberg: Springer Verlag.

Landau, R., Auslander, G. K., Werner, S., Shoval, N., & Heinik, J. (2010). Families' and professional caregivers' views of using advanced technology to track people with dementia. *Qualitative Health Research, 20*(3), 409–419.

Landau, R., & Werner, S. (2012). Ethical aspects of using GPS for tracking people with dementia: Recommendations for practice. *International Psychogeriatrics, 24*(3), 358–366.

Lazar, A., Edasis, C., & Piper, A. M. (2017). A Critical Lens on Dementia and Design in HCI. In *Proceedings of the 2017 CHI Conference on Human Factors in Computing Systems – CHI '17* (pp.2175–2188). Denver: ACM Press.

Learner, S. (2013). Care homes urged to get residents online and stop the 'digital divide' becoming a 'digital gulf'. Retrieved on 29 September 2018 from www.carehome.co.uk/news/article.cfm/id/1560123/care-homes-urged-to-get-residents-online-and-stop-the-digital-divide-becoming-a-digital-gulf

Lee, G. Y., Yip, C. C. K., Yu, E. C. S., & Man, D. W. K. (2013). Evaluation of a computer-assisted errorless learning-based memory training program for patients with early Alzheimer's disease in Hong Kong: A pilot study. *Clinical Interventions in Aging, 8,* 623–633.

Lepore, M., Hughes, S., Wiener, J. M., & Gould, E. (2017). *Including People with Dementia and Their Caregivers as Co-Researchers in Studies of Dementia Care and Services.* Retrieved on 23 October 2018 from https://aspe.hhs.gov/basic-report/including-people-dementia-and-their-caregivers-co-researchers-studies-dementia-care-and-services

Leroi, I., Woolham, J., Gathercole, R., Howard, R., *et al.* (2013). Does telecare prolong community living in dementia? A study protocol for a pragmatic, randomized controlled trial. *Trials, 14,* 349.

Leuty, V., Boger, J., Young, L., Hoey, J., & Mihailidis, A. (2013). Engaging older adults with dementia in creative occupations using artificially intelligent assistive technology. *Assistive Technology, 2013*(25), 72–79.

Li, D., Park, H. W., Piao, M., & Ryu, K. H. (2016). The Design and Partial Implementation of the Dementia-Aid Monitoring System Based on Sensor Network and Cloud Computing Platform. In R. Lee (ed.), *Applied Computing and Information Technology* (pp.85–100). Cham: Springer International Publishing.

Lindqvist, E., Larsson, T. J., & Borell, L. (2015). Experienced usability of assistive technology for cognitive support with respect to user goals. *Neurorehabilitation, 36,* 135–149.

Lindqvist, E., Nygård, L., & Borell, L. (2013). Significant junctures on the way towards becoming a user of assistive technology in Alzheimer's disease. *Scandinavian Journal of Occupational Therapy, 20*(5), 386–396.

Lindqvist, E., Persson Vasiliou, A., Hwang, A., Michailidis, A., Sixsmith, A., Astell, A., & Nygård, L. (2016). What everyday activities do people with mild cognitive impairments want to maintain mastery of – and why? *British Journal of Occupational Therapy*, *79*(7), 399–408.

Lindsay, S., Brittain, K., Jackson, D., Ladha, C., Ladha, K., & Olivier, P. (2012). Empathy, participatory design and people with dementia. In *Proceedings of the 2012 ACM Annual Conference on Human Factors in Computing Systems – CHI '12* (pp.521–530). New York: ACM Press.

Lithfous, S., Dufour, A., & Despres, O. (2013). Spatial navigation in normal aging and the prodromal stage of Alzheimer's disease: Insights from imaging and behavioral studies. *Ageing Research Reviews*, *12*(1), 201–213.

Liu, A. L., Hile, H., Kautz, H., Borriello, G., *et al.* (2008). Indoor wayfinding: Developing a functional interface for individuals with cognitive impairments. *Disability and Rehabilitation: Assistive Technology*, *3*(1–2), 69–81.

Liu, S., Liu, S., Cai, W., Pujol, S., Kikinis, R., & Feng, D. (2014). Early Diagnosis of Alzheimer's Disease with Deep Learning. Paper presented at the 2014 IEEE 11th International Symposium on Biomedical Imaging (ISBI), Beijing, China, 29 April–2 May.

Lopez, D., Callen, B., Tirado, F., & Domenech, M. (2009). How to Become a Guardian Angel: Providing Safety in a Home Telecare Service. In A. Mol, I. Moser, & J. Pols (eds), *Care in Practice: On Tinkering in Clinics, Homes and Farms*. Bielefeld: Transcript Verlag.

Lopez-Gomez, D. (2015). Little arrangements that matter: Rethinking autonomy-enabling innovations for later life. *Technological Forecasting and Social Change*, *93*, 91–101.

Lopez-Gomez, D. & Sanchez-Criado, T. (2009). Dwelling the Telecare home: Place, location and habitability. *Space and Culture*, *12*(3), 343–358.

Lorenz, K., Freddolino, P., Comas-Herrera, A., Knapp, M., & Damant, J. (2017). Technology-based tools and services for people with dementia and carers: Mapping technology onto the dementia care pathway. *Dementia*. https://doi.org/10.1177/1471301217691617

Lotfi, A., Langensiepen, C., Mahmoud, S. M., & Akhlaghinia, M. J. (2012). Smart homes for the elderly dementia sufferers: Identification and prediction of abnormal behavior. *Journal of Ambient Intelligence and Humanized Computing*, *3*, 205–218.

Louie, W. Y. G., Li, J., Vaquero, T., & Nejat, G. (2015). Socially Assistive Robots for Seniors Living in Residential Care Homes: User Requirements and Impressions. In D. Coleman (ed.), *Human–Robot Interactions: Principles, Technologies and Challenges* (pp.75–108). Hauppauge, NY: Nova Science Publishers.

Lui, C., Everingham, J., Warburton, J., Cuthill, M., & Bartlet, H. (2009). What makes a community age-friendly: A review of international literature. *Australasian Journal on Ageing*, *28*(3), 116–121.

Lukkien, D., Suijkerbuijk, S., & Leeuw, L. van der. (2015). *Op zoek naar een bruikbaar GPS-systeem voor mensen met dementie of een verstandelijke beperking.* Retrieved on 28 September 2018 from www.domoticawonenzorg.nl/Site_Domotica/docs/onderzoeksrapport-gps-lokalisatietechnologie.pdf

Lynn, J., Rondon-Sulbaran, J., Quinn, E., Ryan, A., McCormack, B., & Martin, S. A. (2017). Systematic review of electronic assistive technology within supported living environments for people with dementia. *Dementia*. https://doi.org/10.1177/1471301217733649

Lyons, B. E., Austin, D., Seelye, A., Petersen, J., *et al.* (2015). Pervasive computing technologies to continuously assess Alzheimer's disease progression and intervention efficacy. *Frontiers in Aging Neuroscience*, *7*(June). https://doi.org/10.3389/fnagi.2015.00102

MacPherson, S., Bird, M., Anderson, K., Davis, T., & Blair, A. (2009). An art gallery access programme for people with dementia: 'You do it for the moment'. *Aging and Mental Health*, *13*(5), 744–752.

Malinowsky, C., Almkvist, O., Kottorp, A., & Nygård, L. (2010). Ability to manage everyday technology: A comparison of persons with dementia or mild cognitive impairment and older adults without cognitive impairment. *Disability and Rehabilitation: Assistive Technology*, *5*, 462–469.

Malinowsky, C., Kottorp, A., & Nygård, L. (2013). Everyday technologies' levels of difficulty when used by older adults with and without cognitive impairment: Comparison of self-perceived versus observed difficulty estimates. *Technology and Disability 25*(3), 167–176.

Malinowsky, C., Nygård, L., & Kottorp, A. (2011). Psychometric evaluation of a new assessment of the ability to manage technology in everyday life. *Scandinavian Journal of Occupational Therapy, 18*, 26–35.

Manera, V., Petit, P.-D. D., Derreumaux, A., Orvieto, I., *et al.* (2015). 'Kitchen and cooking,' a serious game for mild cognitive impairment and Alzheimer's disease: A pilot study. *Frontiers in Aging Neuroscience, 7*(24), 1–10.

Mao, H.-F., Chang, L.-H., Yao, G., Chen, W.-Y., & Huang, W.-N. W. (2015). Indicators of perceived useful dementia care assistive technology: Caregivers' perspectives. *Geriatrics and Gerontology International, 15*(8), 1049–1057.

Marjanovic, S., Lichten, C. A., Robin, E., Parks, S., *et al.* (2016). How policy can help develop and sustain workforce capacity in UK dementia research: Insights from a career tracking analysis and stakeholder interviews. *BMJ Open, 6*(8), e012052.

Marshall, M. (ed.) (2000). *Astrid: A Social and Technological Response to Meeting the Needs of Individuals with Dementia and Their Carers.* London: Hawker Publications.

Martin, L. H., Gutman, H., & Hutton, P.H. (1988). *Technologies of the Self: A Seminar with Michel Foucault.* London: Tavistock.

Martin, R. L. (2009). *The Design of Business: Why Design Thinking is the Next Competitive Advantage.* Boston, MA: Harvard Business Press.

Martin, S., Bengtsson, J. H., & Dröes, R. M. (2010). Assistive Technologies and Issues Relating to Privacy, Ethics and Security. In M. D. Mulvenna, & C. D. Nugent (eds), *Supporting People with Dementia Using Pervasive Health Technologies, Advanced Information and Knowledge Processing* (pp.63–76). London: Springer-Verlag.

Martin, S., Nugent, C., Wallace, J., Kernohan, G., McCreight, B., & Mulvenna, M. (2007). Using context awareness in the 'Smart home' environment to support social care for adults with dementia. *Technology and Disability, 19*(2–3), 143–152.

Marziali, E. & Donahue, P. (2006). Caring for others: Internet video-conferencing group intervention for family caregivers of older adults with neurodegenerative disease. *The Gerontolgist, 46*(3), 398–403.

Marziali, E. & Garcia, L. J. (2011). Dementia caregivers' responses to 2 internet-based intervention programs. *American Journal of Alzheimer's Disease and Other Dementias, 26*(1), 36–43.

Maslow, A. H. (1943). A theory of human motivation. *Psychological Review, 50*(4), 370–396.

Mathias, J. S., Agrawal, A., Feinglass, J., Cooper, A. J., Baker, D. W., & Choudhary, A. (2013). Development of a 5 year life expectancy index in older adults using predictive mining of electronic health record data. *Journal of the American Medical Informatics Association, 20*(e1), e118–e124.

Mathotaarachchi, S., Pascoal, T. A., Shin, M., Benedet, A. L., *et al.* (2017). Identifying incipient dementia individuals using machine learning and amyloid imaging. *Neurobiology of Aging, 59*, 80–90.

McCabe, L. & Innes, A. (2013). Supporting safe walking for people with dementia: User participation in the development of new technology. *Gerontechnology, 12*(1), 4–15.

McColl, D., Chan, J., & Nejat, G. (2012). A socially assistive robot for meal-time cognitive interventions. *Journal of Medical Devices, 6*(1), 017559.

McConatha, D., McConatha, J. T., & Dermigny, R. (1994). The use of interactive computer services to enhance the quality of life for long-term care residents. *Gerontologist, 34*(4), 553–556.

McGoldrick, C. (2017). *MindMate: A single case experimental design study of a reminder system for people with dementia.* D Clin Psy thesis, University of Glasgow.

McShane, R., Gedling, K., Kenward, B., Kenward, R., Hope, T., & Jacoby, R. (1998). The feasibility of electronic tracking devices in dementia: A telephone survey and case series. *International Journal of Geriatric Psychiatry*, *13*(8), 556–563.

Medium. (2017). *Using the Amazon Echo to improve the lives of Alzheimer's patients*. Retrieved on 30 September 2018 from https://medium.com/@JaysThoughts/using-the-amazon-echo-to-improve-the-lives-of-alzheimers-patients-f5727560a5eb

Megges, H., Freiesleben, S., Jankowski, N., Haas, B., & Peters, O. (2017). Technology for home dementia care: A prototype locating system put to the test. *Alzheimer's and Dementia: Translational Research and Clinical Interventions*, *3*(3), 332–338.

Meiland, F., Innes, A., Mountain, G., Robinson, L., *et al.* (2017). Technologies to support community-dwelling persons with dementia: A position paper on issues regarding development, usability, effectiveness and cost-effectiveness, deployment, and ethics. *JMIR Rehabilitation and Assistive Technologies*, *4*(1), e1.

Merriam-Webster. (2018). *Artificial intelligence*. Retrieved on 7 October 2018 from www.merriam-webster.com/dictionary/artificial%20intelligence

Microsoft. (2010). Windows Azure General Availability. *The Official Microsoft Blog*. Retrieved on 7 October 2018 from https://blogs.microsoft.com/blog/2010/02/01/windows-azure-general-availability

Mihailidis, A. (2017). *Ubiquitous Robotics to Support Older Adults with Dementia*. Retrieved on 28 September 2018 from http://iatsl.org/projects/ubiquitous_robotics.html

Mihailidis, A., Barbenel, J. C., & Fernie, G. (2004). The efficacy of an intelligent cognitive orthosis to facilitate handwashing by persons with moderate to severe dementia. *Neuropsychological Rehabilitation*. https://doi.org/10.1080/09602010343000156

Milligan, C., Roberts, C., & Mort, M. (2011). Telecare and older people: Who cares where? *Social Science and Medicine*, *72*(3), 347–354.

Mitchell, T. M. (1997). *Machine Learning*. New York: McGraw-Hill Education.

MOPEAD. (2016). *RUN 1 AD CItizen Science*. Retrieved on 28 September 2018 from www.mopead.eu/single-post/RUN1-AD-CItizen-Science

Morgan, D., Crossley, M., Stewart, N., Kirk, A., *et al.* (2014). Evolution of a community-based participatory approach in a rural and remote dementia care research program. *Progress in Community Health Partnerships*, *8*(3), 337–345.

Morgan, J. (2016). Gaming for dementia research: A quest to save the brain. *The Lancet Neurology*, *15*(13), 1313.

Morris, R. G., Downes, J. J., Sahakian, B. J., Evenden, J. L., Heald, A., & Robbins, T. W. (1988). Planning and spatial working memory in Parkinson's disease. *Journal of Neurology, Neurosurgery, and Psychiatry*, *51*(6), 757–766.

Morrissey, K., McCarthy, J., & Pantidi, N. (2017). The Value of Experience-Centred Design Approaches in Dementia Research Contexts. In *Proceedings of the 2017 CHI Conference on Human Factors in Computing Systems – CHI '17* (pp.1326–1338). Denver: ACM Press.

Mort, M., Roberts, C., & Callen, B. (2013). Ageing with telecare: Care or coercion in austerity. *Sociology of Health and Illness*, *35*(6), 799–812.

Mort, M., Roberts, C., Pols, J., Domenech, M., & Moser, I. (2015). Ethical implications of home telecare for older people: A framework derived from a multisited participative study. *Health Expectations*, *18*(3), 438–449.

Mountain, G. A., & Craig, C. L. (2012). What should be in a self-management programme for people with early dementia? *Ageing and Mental Health*, *16*(5), 576–583.

Moyle, W., Jones, C., Dwan, T., & Petrovich, T. (2017). Effectiveness of a virtual reality forest on people with dementia: A mixed methods pilot study. *The Gerontologist*. https://doi.org/10.1093/geront/gnw270

Muller, M. J. (2003). Participatory design: The third space in HCI. *Human–Computer Interaction Handbook*, *4235*, 1051–1068.

Müller-Rakow, A. & Flechtner, R. (2017). Designing interactive music systems with and for people with dementia. *The Design Journal, 20*(supp.1), S2207–S2214.

National Center for Complementary and Intergrative Health. (2018). *Finding and Evalauating Online Sources.* Retrieved on 28 September 2018 from https://nccih.nih.gov/health/webresources

National Museums Liverpool. (2012). *House of Memories. An Evaluation of National Museums Liverpool: Dementia Training Programme, May 2012.* Retrieved on 30 September 2018 from www.liverpoolmuseums.org.uk/learning/documents/house-of-memories-evaluation-report.pdf

Neubauer, N., Fernandez, V., Liu, L., & Stroulia, E. (2018). Effect of Kinect Tai Chi on overall health of dementia clients: A feasibility and usability study. *Innovation in Ageing, 1*(May), 661–662.

Newbronner, L., Chamberlain, R., Borthwick, R., Baxter, M., & Glendinning, C. (2013). *A Road Less Rocky: Supporting Carers of People with Dementia.* Retrieved on 28 September 2018 from https://carers.org/sites/default/files/media/dementia_executive_summary_english_only_final_use_this_one.pdf

Newell, A. F., Gregor, P., Morgan, M., Pullin, G., & Macaulay, C. (2011). User-sensitive inclusive design. *Universal Access in the Information Society, 10*(3), 235–243.

Newton, L., Dickinson, C., Gibson, G., Brittain, K., & Robinson, L. (2016). Exploring the views of GPs, people with dementia and their carers on assistive technology: A qualitative study. *BMJ Open, 6,* e011132.

NHS Choices. (2015). *Become a Confident Internet User.* Retrieved on 28 September 2018 from www.nhs.uk/NHSEngland/digital-inclusion/Pages/get-online-take-control-of-your-health.aspx

Niemeijer, A., Frederiks, B., Depla, M., Eefsting, J., & Hertogh, C. (2013). The place of surveillance technology in residential care for people with intellectual disabilities: Is there an ideal model of application. *Journal of Intellectual Disability Research, 57*(3), 201–215.

Norman, D., Miller, J., & Henderson, A. (1995). What You See, Some of What's in the Future, And How We Go About Doing It: HI at Apple Computer. In *Proceedings of the 1995 CHI Conference on Human Factors in Computing Systems (p.155).* New York: ACM Press.

Noto La Diega, G. & Walden, I. (2016). *Contracting for the 'Internet of Things': Looking into the Nest.* Retrieved on 28 September 2018 from https://ssrn.com/abstract=2725913

Novitzky, P., Smeaton, A., Chen, C., Orving, K., *et al.* (2015). A review of contemporary work on the ethics of ambient assisted living technologies for people with dementia. *Science and Engineering Ethics, 21*(3), 707–765.

Nugent, C. D., Davies, R. J., Donnelly, M. P., Hallberg, J., *et al.* (2008). The development of personalised cognitive prosthetics. In *Conference Proceedings: Annual International Conference of the IEEE Engineering in Medicine and Biology Society. IEEE Engineering in Medicine and Biology Society Conference 2008* (pp.787–790). Vancouver: IEEE.

Nygård, L. (2008). The meaning of everyday technology as experienced by people with dementia who live alone. *Dementia, 7*(4), 481–502.

Nygård, L. (2009). The stove timer as a device for older adults with cognitive impairment or dementia: Different professionals' reasoning and actions. *Technology and Disability, 21,* 53–66.

Nygård, L., Borell, L., & Gustavsson, A. (1995). Managing images of occupational self in early stage dementia. *Scandinavian Journal of Occupational Therapy, 2,* 129–137.

Nygård, L. & Johansson, M. (2001). The experience and management of temporality in five cases of dementia. *Scandinavian Journal of Occupational Therapy, 8,* 85–95.

Nygård, L., Pantzar, M., Uppgard, B., & Kottorp, A. (2012). Detection of disability in older adults with MCI or Alzheimer's disease through assessment of perceived difficulty in using everyday technology. *Aging and Mental Health, 16*(3–4), 361–371.

Nygård, L. & Rosenberg, L. (2016). How attention to everyday technology could contribute to modern occupational therapy: A focus group study. *British Journal of Occupational Therapy*, *79*(8), 467–474.

Nygård, L. & Starkhammar, S. (2007). The use of everyday technology by people with dementia living alone. *Aging and Mental Health*, *11*(2), 144–155.

Nygård, L., Starkhammar, S., & Lilja, M. (2008). The provision of stove timers to individuals with cognitive impairment. *Scandinavian Journal of Occupational Therapy*, *15*, 4–12.

OED Online. (2017). Citizen science. *Oxford English Dictionary*. Oxford: Oxford University Press.

Oldman, C. (2003). Deceiving, theorizing and self-justification: A critique of independent living. *Critical Social Policy*, *23*(1), 44–62.

Oliver, K. (2016). *Walk the Walk, Talk the Talk*. Kent: Forget-Me-Nots.

Oliver, K. (2019) *Dear Alzheimer's*. London: Jessica Kingsley Publishers.

Onoda, K., Hamano, T., Nabika, Y., Aoyama, A., *et al.* (2013). Validation of a new mass screening tool for cognitive impairment: Cognitive assessment for dementia, iPad version. *Clinical Interventions in Aging*, *8*, 353–360.

Orpwood, R., Adlam, T., Evans, N., Chadd, J., & Self, D. (2008). Evaluation of an assisted-living smart home for someone with dementia. *Journal of Assistive Technologies*, *2*(2), 13–21.

Orpwood, R., Chadd, J., Howcroft, D., Sixsmith, A., *et al.* (2010). Designing technology to improve quality of life for people with dementia: User led approaches. *Universal Access in the Information Society*, *9*(3), 249–259.

Orpwood, R., Gibbs, C., Adlam, T., Faulkner, R., & Meegahawatte, D. (2004). The Gloucester Smart House for People with Dementia—User-Interface Aspects. In S. Keates, J. Clarkson, & P. Langdon (eds), *Designing a More Inclusive World* (pp.237–245). London: Springer.

Orpwood, R., Gibbs, C., Adlam, T., Faulkner, R., & Meegahawatte, D. (2005). The design of smart homes for people with dementia – user-interface aspects. *Universal Access in the Information Society*, *4*(2), 156–164.

Orpwood, R., Sixsmith, A., Torrington, J., Chadd, J., Gibson, G., & Chalfont, G. (2007). Designing technology to support quality of life of people with dementia. *Technology and Disability*, *19*(2–3), 103–112.

Osman, S. E., Tischler, V., & Schneider, J. (2016). 'Singing for the Brain': A qualitative study exploring the health and well-being benefits of singing for people with dementia and their carers. *Dementia*, *15*(6), 1326–1339.

Östlund, B. (2010). Watching television in later life: A deeper understanding of TV viewing in the homes of old people and in geriatric care contexts. *Scandinavian Journal of Caring Sciences*, *24*(2), 233–243.

Palm, E., & Hansson, S. O. (2006) The case for ethical technology assessment. *Technological Forecasting and Social Change*, *73*, 543–558.

Passini, R., Rainville, C., Marchand, N., & Joanette, Y. (1995). Wayfinding in dementia of the Alzheimer type: Planning abilities. *Journal of Clinical and Experimental Neuropsychology*. https://doi.org/10.1080/01688639508402431

Passini, R., Rainville, C., Marchand, N., & Joanette, Y. (1998). Wayfinding and dementia: Some research findings and a new look at design. *Journal of Architectural and Planning Research*, *15*, 133–151.

Pearson, S. & Benameur, A. (2010). Privacy, Security and Trust Issues Arising from Cloud Computing. *2nd IEEE International Conference on Cloud Computing Technology and Science* (pp.693–702). Washington, DC: IEEE Computer Society.

Percival, J. & Hanson, J. (2006). Big brother or brave new world? Telecare and its implications for older people's independence and social inclusion. *Critical Social Policy*, *26*(4), 888–909.

Perry, J., Beyer, S., & Holm, S. (2009). Assistive technology, telecare and people with intellectual disabilities: Ethical considerations. *Journal of Medical Ethics*, *35*, 81–86.

Phillips, L. J., Reid-Arndt, S., & Pak, Y. (2010). Effects of a creative expression intervention on emotions, communication, and quality of life in persons with dementia. *Nursing Research*, *59*(6), 417–425.

Phillipson, L., Hall, D., Cridland, E., Fleming, R., *et al.* (2018). Involvement of people with dementia in raising awareness and changing attitudes in a dementia friendly community pilot project. *Dementia*. https://doi.org/10.1177/1471301218754455

PhRMA. (2015). *Alzheimer's Medicines: Setbacks and Stepping Stones.* Retrieved on 28 September 2018 from www.phrma.org/report/researching-alzheimer-s-medicines-setbacks-and-stepping-stones

Pineau, J., Montemerlo, M., Pollack, M., Roy, N., & Thrun, S. (2003). Towards robotic assistants in nursing homes: Challenges and results. In *Robotics and Autonomous Systems*, *42*, 271–281.

Pini, S., Ingleson, E., Megson, M., Clare, L., Wright, P., & Oyebode, J. R. (2018). A needs-led framework for understanding the impact of caring for a family member with dementia. *The Gerontologist*, *58*(2), e68–e77.

Playlist for Life (n.d.) *Research Findings.* Retrieved on 28 September 2018 from www.playlistforlife. org.uk/Handlers/Download.ashx?IDMF=613e2f38-867e-40ef-9bc4-7b233a625439

Pols, J. & Moser, I. (2009). Cold technologies versus warm care? On affective and social relations with and through care technologies. *ALTER European Journal of Disability Research*, *3*(2), 159–178.

Prensky, M. (2001). Digital natives, digital immigrants: Part 1. *On the Horizon*, *9*(5), 1–6.

President and Fellows of Harvard College. (2017). *What Is STS?* Retrieved on 28 September 2018 from http://sts.hks.harvard.edu/about/whatissts.html

Procter, R., Wherton, J., Greenhalgh, T., Sugarhood, P., Rouncefield, M., & Hinder, S. (2016). Telecare call centre work and ageing in place. *Computer Supported Cooperative Work*, *25*(1), 79–105.

Puran, N. (2005). Ulysses Contracts: Bound to treatment or free to choose? *The York Scholar*, *2*, 42–51.

Purves, B. A., Phinney, A., Hulko, W., Puurveen, G., & Astell, A. J. (2015). Developing CIRCA-BC and exploring the role of the computer as a third participant in conversation. *American Journal of Alzheimer's Disease and Other Dementias*, *30*(1), 101–107.

Quaglio, G., Corbetta, M., Karapiperis, T., *et al.* (2017). Understanding the brain through large, multidisciplinary research initiatives. *The Lancet*, *16*(3), 183–184.

Richards, D. (2017). *Using big data to fight dementia.* Retrieved on 28 September 2018 from www.huffingtonpost.co.uk/david-richards/using-big-data-to-fight-d_b_15961386.html

Riesch, H. & Potter, C. (2013). Citizen science as seen by scientists: Methodological, epistemological and ethical dimensions. *Public Understanding of Science*, *23*(1), 107–120.

Riley, P., Alm, N., & Newell, A. (2009). An interactive tool to promote musical creativity in people with dementia. *Computers in Human Behavior*, *25*(3), 599–608.

Ritchie, K., Allard, M., Huppert, F. A., Nargeot, C., Pinek, B., & Ledesert, B. (1993). Computerized cognitive examination of the elderly (ECO): The development of a neuropsychological examination for clinic and population use. *International Journal of Geriatric Psychiatry*, *8*(11), 899–914.

Robbins, T. W., James, M., Owen, A. M., Sahakian, B. J., McInnes, L., & Rabbitt, P. (1994). Cambridge Neuropsychological Test Automated Battery (CANTAB): A factor analytic study of a large sample of normal elderly volunteers. *Dementia*, *5*(5), 266–281.

Roberts, V., Mort, M., & Milligan, C. (2012). Calling for care: 'Disembodied' work, teleoperators and older people living at home. *Sociology*, *46*(3), 490–506.

Robertson, T. & Simonsen, J. (2013). Participatory Design. An introduction. In T. Robertson & J. Simonsen (eds), *Routledge International Handbook of Participatory Design* (pp. 1–17). Abingdon: Routledge.

Robinson, L., Brittain, K., Lindsay, S., Jackson, D., & Olivier, P. (2009). Keeping In Touch Everyday (KITE) project: Developing assistive technologies with people with dementia and their carers to promote independence. *International Psychogeriatrics, 21*(3), 494–502.

Robinson, L., Hutchings, D., Corner, L., Finch, T., *et al.* (2007). Balancing rights and risks: Conflicting perspectives in the management of wandering in dementia. *Health, Risk and Society, 9*(4), 389–406.

Rosenberg, L., Kottorp, A., & Nygård, L. (2012). Readiness for technology use with people with dementia: Views of significant others. *Journal of Applied Gerontology, 31*(4), 510–530.

Rosenberg, L. & Nygård, L. (2010). *Teknik som stöd för personer med demens och deras närstående.* (Technology as support for people with dementia and their families). Stockholm: Hjälpmedelsinstitutet (Swedish Handicap Institute).

Rosenberg, L. & Nygård, L. (2012). Persons with dementia become users of assistive technology: A study of the process. *Dementia, 11*(2), 135–154.

Rosenberg, L. & Nygård, L. (2014). Learning and using technology in intertwined processes: A study of people with MCI/AD. *Dementia, 13*(5), 662–677.

Rosenberg, L. & Nygård, L. (2017). Learning and knowing technology as lived experience in people with Alzheimer's disease: A phenomenological study. *Ageing and Mental Health, 21*(12), 1272–1279.

Rosenberg, L., Nygård, L., & Kottorp, A. (2009). Everyday Technology Use Questionnaire (ETUQ): Evaluation of the psychometric properties of a new assessment of competence in technology use. *Occupational Therapy Journal of Research, 29*(2), 52–62.

Roy, N., Baltus, G., Fox, D., Gemperle, F., *et al.* (2000). Towards Personal Service Robots for the Elderly. *Workshop on Interactive Robots and Entertainment (WIRE 2000), 25,* 184.

Rubin, J. (1994) *Handbook of Usability, How to Plan, Design and Conduct Effective Tests.* New York: John Wiley & Sons.

Rubinstein, E., Duggan, C., Van Landingham, B., Thompson, D., & Warburton, W. (2015). *A Call to Action: The Global Response to Dementia Through Policy Innovation.* Retrieved on 28 September 2018 from www.wish.org.qa/wp-content/uploads/2018/01/WISH_Dementia_Forum_Report_08.01.15_WEB.pdf

Ruckriem, G. (2009). Digital technology and mediation: A challenge to activity theory. In A. Sannino, H. Daniels, & K. D. Gutiérrez (eds), *Learning and Expanding with Activity Theory.* Cambridge: Cambridge University Press.

Sahakian, B. J., Morris, R. G., Evenden, J. L., Heald, A., *et al.* (1988). A comparative study of visuospatial memory and learning in Alzheimer-type dementia and Parkinson's disease. *Brain, 111*(Pt 3), 695–718.

Samuel, A. L. (1959). Some studies in machine learning using the game of checkers. *IBM Journal of Research and Development, 3*(3), 210–229.

Sandberg, L., Rosenberg, L., Sandman, P.-O., and Borell, L. (2017). Risks in situations that are experienced as unfamiliar and confusing: The perspective of persons with dementia. *Dementia, 16*(4), 471–485.

Sanders, E. & Stappers, P. J. (2008). Co-creation and the new landscapes of design. *CoDesign, 4*(1), 5–18.

Savenstedt, S., Brulin, C., & Sandman, P.-O. (2003). Family members' narrated experiences of communicating via video-phone with patients with dementia staying at a nursing home. *Journal of Telemedicine and Telecare, 9*(4), 216–220.

Savitch, N., Brooks D., and Wey, S. (2012). AT Guide: Developing a new way to help people with dementia and their carers find information about assistive technology. *Journal of Assistive Technologies, 6*(1), 76–80.

Savitch, N. & Zaphiris, P. (2007). Web Site Design for People with Dementia. In S. Kurniawan & P. Zaphiris (eds), *Advances in Universal Web Design and Evaluation* (pp.220–256). London: Idea Group.

Schikhof, Y. & Wauben, L. (2016). Virtual cycling for people with dementia. *Gerontechnology*, *15*(163). https://doi.org/10.4017/gt.2016.15.s.709.00

Schols, J. & Kardol, T. (2017). Dementia Care in Nursing Homes Requires a Multidisciplinary Approach. In S. Schüssler, & C. Lohrmann (eds), *Dementia in Nursing Homes* (pp.203–217). Cham: Springer International Publishing.

Schölzel-Dorenbos, C. J., Meeuwsen, E. J., and Olde Rikkert, M. G. (2010). Integrating unmet needs into dementia health-related quality of life research and care: Introduction of the Hierarchy Model of Needs in Dementia. *Aging and Mental Health*, *14*(1), 113–119.

Schreiber, M., Schweizer, A., Lutz, K., Kalveram, K. T., & Jäncke, L. (1999). Potential of an interactive computer-based training in the rehabilitation of dementia: An initial study. *Neuropsychological Rehabilitation*, *9*(2), 155–167.

Schroeder, R. (2014). Big data and the brave new world of social media research. *Big Data and Society*, *1*(2), 2053951714563194.

Scottish Dementia Working Group. (2013). *Core Principles for Involving People with Dementia in Research*. Retrieved on 28 September 2018 from https://coreprinciplesdementia.wordpress.com

Scottish Government. (2017). *Scotland's National Dementia Strategy 2017–2020*. Edinburgh: Scottish Government.

Seale, J. (2014). The role of supporters in facilitating the use of technologies by adolescents and adults with learning disabilities: A place for positive risk-taking? *European Journal of Special Needs Education*, *29*(2), 220–236.

Seale, J. & Chadwick, D. (2017). How does risk mediate the ability of adolescents and adults with intellectual and developmental disabilities to live a normal life by using the Internet? *Cyberpsychology: Journal of Psychosocial Research on Cyberspace*, *11*(1), article 2. http://dx.doi.org/10.5817/CP2017-1-2

Seixas, F. L., Zadrozny, B., Laks, J., Conci, A., & Muchaluat Saade, D. C. (2014). A Bayesian network decision model for supporting the diagnosis of dementia, Alzheimer's disease and mild cognitive impairment. *Computers in Biology and Medicine*, *51*(Supplement C), 140–158.

Selwyn, N., Gorard, S., Furlong, J., & Madden, L. (2003). Older adults' use of information and communications technology in everyday life. *Ageing and Society*, *23*(5), 561–582.

Sempik, J., Aldridge, J., & and Becker, S. (2002) *Social and Therapeutic Horticulture: Evidence and Messages from Research*. Reading: Thrive (in association with the Centre for Child and Family Research).

Sharkey, A. & Sharkey, N. (2014). Granny and the robots: Ethical issues in robot care for the elderly. *Ethics and Information Technology*, *14*(1), 27–40.

Sheehan, B., Burton, E., & Mitchell, L. (2006). Outdoor wayfinding in dementia. *Dementia*, *5*(2), 271–281.

Shen, L., Kennedy, D., & Preuss, N. (2013). The three NITRCs: Software, data and cloud computing for brain science and dementia research. *Alzheimer's and Dementia: The Journal of the Alzheimer's Association*, *9*(4), 255–256.

Shin, D., Shin, D., & Shin, D. (2014). Ubiquitous health management system with watch-type monitoring device for dementia patients. *Journal of Applied Mathematics*, 8. doi:10.1155/2014/878741

Silverstein, M. & Parker, M. G. (2002). Leisure activities and quality of life among the oldest old in Sweden. *Research on Aging*, *24*(5), 528–547.

Simonsick, E. M., Guralnik, J. M., Volpato, S., Balfour, J., & Fried, L. P. (2005). Just get out the door! Importance of walking outside the home for maintaining mobility: Findings from the Women's Health and Aging Study. *Journal of the American Geriatrics Society*, *53*(2), 198–203.

Singer, P. (2011). *The Expanding Circle: Ethics, Evolution, and Moral Progress*. Princeton, NJ: Princeton University Press.

Sixsmith, A. & Gibson, G. (2007). Music and the wellbeing of people with dementia. *Ageing and Society*, *27*(1), 127–145.

Sixsmith, A. & Sixsmith, J. (2008). Ageing in place in the United Kingdom. *Ageing International*, *32*(3), 219–235.

Smaradottir, B. F., Martinez, S., Holen-Rabbersvik, E., & Fensli, R. (2015). eHealth-Extended Care Coordination: Development of a Collaborative System for Inter-municipal Dementia Teams: A Research Project with a User-Centered Design Approach. Paper presented at the 2015 International Conference on Computational Science and Computational Intelligence (CSCI), Las Vegas, Nevada, 7–9 December.

Smebye, K. L., Kirkevold, M., & Engedal, K. (2016). Ethical dilemmas concerning autonomy when persons with dementia wish to live at home: A qualitative, hermeneutic study. *BMC Health Services Research*, *16*(21). https://doi.org/10.1186/s12913-015-1217-1

Smith, G. E. (2013). Everyday technologies across the continuum of dementia care. In *Conference Proceedings: Annual International Conference of the IEEE Engineering in Medicine and Biology Society. IEEE Engineering in Medicine and Biology Society Conference 2013* (pp.7040–7043). Vancouver: IEEE.

Smith, S. K. (2015). *Exploring the potential of touch-screen computer technology in promoting enjoyable activities for people living with dementia: A visual ethnography*. PhD thesis, University of Sheffield, Faculty of Medicine, Dentistry and Health, School of Health and Related Research, Sheffield.

Smith, S. K. & Mountain, G. A. (2012). New forms of information and communication technology (ICT) and the potential to facilitate social and leisure activity for people living with dementia. *International Journal of Computers in Healthcare*, *1*(4), 332.

Social Care Institute for Excellence. (2017). Using Technology to Support People with Dementia. Retrieved on 28 September 2018 from www.scie.org.uk/dementia/support/technology

Span, M., Hettinga, M., Vernooij-Dassen, M., Eefsting, J., & Smits, C. (2013). Involving people with dementia in the development of supportive IT applications: A systematic review. *Ageing Research Reviews*, *12*(2), 535–551.

Sposaro, F., Danielson, J., & Tyson, G. (2010). IWander: An Android application for dementia patients. In *Conference Proceedings: Annual International Conference of the IEEE Engineering in Medicine and Biology Society. IEEE Engineering in Medicine and Biology Society Conference 2010* (pp.3875–3878). Vancouver: IEEE.

Starkhammar, S. and Nygård, L. (2008). Using a timer device for the stove: Experiences of older adults with memory impairment or dementia and their families. *Technology and Disability*, *20*, 189–191.

Statista. (2017). *Number of Available Apps from the iTunes App Store 2008–2017*. Retrieved on 2 May 2018 from www.statista.com/statistics/268251/number-of-apps-in-the-itunes-app-store-since-2008

Steventon, A., Bardsley, M., Billings, J., Dixon, J., Doll, H., & Beynon, M. (2013). Effect of telecare on use of health and social care services: Findings from the Whole Systems Demonstrator cluster randomised trial. *Age and Ageing*, *42*(4), 501–508.

Stock, S. E., Davies, D. K., Wehmeyer, M. L., & Lachapelle, Y. (2011). Emerging new practices in technology to support independent community access for people with intellectual and cognitive disabilities. *NeuroRehabilitation*, *28*, 261–269.

Stokes, V. & Savitch, N (2011). *We Can Do IT Too: Using Computers in Activity Programmes for People with Dementia*. Oxford: Routledge

STS Wiki. (2010). *Welcome to the Worldwide Directory of STS Programs!* Retrieved on 28 September 2018 from http://stswiki.org/index.php?title=Worldwide_directory_of_STS_programs

Stuss, D. T., Amira, S., Rossor, M., Johnson, R., & Khachaturian, Z. (2015). How We Can Work Together on Research and Health Big Data: Strategies to Ensure Value and Success. In G. Anderson & J. Oderkirk (eds), *Dementia Research and Care: Can Big Data Help?* (pp.61–75). Paris: OECD Publishing.

Suijkerbuijk, S., Brankaert, R., de Kort, Y. A. W., Snaphaan, Li., & den Ouden, E. (2015). Seeing the first-person perspective in dementia: A qualitative personal evaluation game to evaluate assistive technology for people affected by dementia in the home context. *Interacting with Computers*, *27*(1), 47–59.

Suijkerbuijk, S., Cornelisse, C. C., van der Leeuw, J., & Nap, H. H. (2016). User evaluation of a navigation application for people with mild cognitive impairment (MCI): A two months test in the Netherlands and Spain. *Gerontechnology*, *15*(suppl.), 117.

SV Health Managers LLP. (n.d.). *Dementia Discovery Fund.* Retrieved on 28 September 2018 from http://theddfund.com

Tan, Z. S., Damron-Rodriguez, J., Cadogan, M., Gans, D., *et al.* (2017). Team-based interprofessional competency training for dementia screening and management. *Journal of the American Geriatrics Society*, *65*(1), 207–211.

Tandon, R., Adak, S., & Kaye, J. A. (2006). Neural networks for longitudinal studies in Alzheimer's disease. *Artificial Intelligence in Medicine*, *36*(3), 245–255.

Tesler, L. (2018). *Adages & Coinages.* Retrieved from http://www.udu.co/blog/whatever-machines-havent-done-yet

The World Bank & International Monetary Fund. (2016). *Global Monitoring Report 2015/2016: Development Goals in an Era of Demographic Change.* Washington, DC: World Bank. Retrieved on 28 September 2018 from http://pubdocs.worldbank.org/en/503001444058224597/Global-Monitoring-Report-2015.pdf

Thelen, B. A. & Thiet, R. K. (2008). Cultivating connection: Incorporating meaningful citizen science into Cape Cod National Seashore's estuarine research and monitoring programs. *Park Science*, *25*(1), 74–80.

Thompson, R. (2017). *Guidance for Using the Life Story Book Template.* London: Dementia UK. Retrieved on 23 October 2018 from www.dementiauk.org/wp-content/uploads/2017/03/Lifestory-.compressed.pdf

Thompson Klein, J. (2004). Prospects for transdisciplinarity. *Futures*, *36*(4), 515–526.

Thorpe, J. R., Rønn-Andersen, K. V. H., Bień, P., Özkil, A. G., Forchhammer, B. H., & Maier, A. M. (2016). Pervasive assistive technology for people with dementia: A UCD case. *Healthcare Technology Letters*, *3*(4), 297–302.

Tinder Foundation. (2016). *Dementia and Digital: Using Technology to Improve Health and Wellbeing for People with Dementia and Their Carers.* Retrieved on 28 September 2018 from www.goodthingsfoundation.org/sites/default/files/research-publications/dementia_and_digital.pdf

Toot, S., Hoe, J., Ledgerd, R., Burnell K., Devine, M., & Orrell, M. (2013). Causes of crises and appropriate interventions: The views of people with dementia, carers and healthcare professionals. *Aging and Mental Health*, *17*(3), 328–335.

Topo, P. (2009). Technology studies to meet the needs of people with dementia and their caregivers: A literature review. *Journal of Applied Gerontology*, *28*(1), 5–37.

Treadaway, C. & Kenning, G. (2016). Sensor e-textiles: Person centered co-design for people with late stage dementia. *Working with Older People*, *20*(2), 76–85.

Twedt, E., Proffitt, D. R., & Hearn, D. L. (2014). Art and aging: Digital projects for individuals with dementia. *Journal of Social and Political Psychology*, *2*(1), 61–70.

Tyack, C. & Camic, P. M. (2017). Touchscreen interventions and the well-being of people with dementia and caregivers: A systematic review. *International Psychogeriatrics*, *29*(8), 1261–1280.

Uc, E. Y., Rizzo, M., Anderson, S. W., Shi, Q., & Dawson, J. D. (2004). Driver route-following and safety errors in early Alzheimer disease. *Neurology*, *65*(5), 832–837.

University of Alberta. (2017). *Science, Technology and Society.* Retrieved on 28 September 2018 from www.ualberta.ca/interdisciplinary-studies/science-technology-and-society

University of Oxford for the Oxford Internet Institute. (2014). *Big Data for Advancing Dementia Research.* Retrieved on 28 September 2018 from http://bigdatadementia.oii.ox.ac.uk

van Kooten, J., Delwel, S., Binnekade, T. T., Smalbrugge, M., *et al.* (2015). Pain in dementia: Prevalence and associated factors: Protocol of a multidisciplinary study. *BMC Geriatrics*, *15*(1), 29.

van Rest, J., Boonstra, D., Everts, M., van Rijn, M., & van Paassen, R. (2012). Designing privacy-by-design. Presented at Privacy Technologies and Policy, First Annual Privacy Forum 2012, Limassol, Cyprus, 10–11 October.

Verhoeven, F., Cremers, A., Schoone, M., & van Dijk, J. (2016). Mobiles for mobility: Participatory design of a 'Happy Walker' that stimulates mobility among older people. *Gerontechnology*, *15*(1), 32–44.

Wallace, J., Wright, P. C., McCarthy, J., Green, D. P., Thomas, J., & Olivier, P. (2013). A design-led inquiry into personhood in dementia. In *Extended Abstracts on Human Factors in Computing Systems – CHI EA '13* (pp.2883–2884). New York: ACM Press.

Wan, L., Müller, C., Randall, D., & Wulf, V. (2016). Design of a GPS monitoring system for dementia care and its challenges in academia-industry project. *ACM Transactions on Computer–Human Interaction*, *23*(5), 1–36.

Wandke, H., Sengpiel, M., & Sönksen, M. (2012). Myths about older people's use of information and communication technology. *Gerontology*, *58*(6), 564–570.

Watts, P. (2017). Forget-me-nots in Purley: How the town became 'dementia friendly'. *The Guardian*, 2 February. Retrieved on 30 September 2018 from www.theguardian.com/cities/2017/feb/02/purley-uk-latest-dementia-friendly-community

Weir, A. J., Paterson, C. A., Tieges, Z., MacLullich, A. M., *et al.* (2014). Development of Android apps for cognitive assessment of dementia and delirium. In *36th Annual International Conference of the IEEE Engineering in Medicine and Biology Society* (pp.2169–2172). Vancouver: IEEE.

Wherton, J. & Monk, A. (2008). Technological opportunities for supporting people with dementia who are living at home. *International Journal of Human–Computer Studies*, *66*(8), 571–586.

Whitebird, R. R., Kreitzer, M. J., Crain, A. L., Lewis, B. A., Hanson, L. R., & Enstad, C. J. (2013). Mindfulness-based stress reduction for family caregivers: A randomized controlled trial. *The Gerontologist*, *53*(4), 676–686.

Wilcock, A. (1999). Reflections on doing, being and becoming. *Australian Occupational Therapy Journal*, *46*, 1–11.

Wilson, J. & Rosenberg, D. (1988). Rapid Prototyping for User Interface Design. In G. Helander (ed.), *Handbook of Human–Computer Interaction* (pp.859–875). Amsterdam: Elsevier.

Woolham, J., Gibson, G., & Clarke, P. (2006). Assistive technology, telecare and dementia: Some implications of current policies and guidance. *Research Policy and Planning*, *24*, 149–164.

World Health Organization. (2017). *Draft Global Action Plan on the Public Health Response to Dementia*. Retrieved on 28 September 2018 from http://apps.who.int/gb/ebwha/pdf_files/EB140/B140_28-en.pdf?ua=1

Yaw-Jen, L., Heng-Shuen, C., & Mei-Ju, S. (2015). A Cloud Based Bluetooth Low Energy Tracking System for Dementia Patients. Paper presented at the Eighth International Conference on Mobile Computing and Ubiquitous Networking (ICMU), Hakodate, Japan, 20–22 January.

Ye, J., Farnum, M., Yang, E., Verbeeck, R., *et al.* (2012). Sparse learning and stability selection for predicting MCI to AD conversion using baseline ADNI data. *BMC Neurology*, *12*(1), 46.

Zheng, J., Chen, X., & Yu, P. (2017). Game-based interventions and their impact on dementia: A narrative review. *Australasian Psychiatry*. https://doi.org/10.1177/1039856217726686

Zwijsen, S., Niemeijer, A., & Hertogh, C. (2011). Ethics of using assistive technology in the care of community-dwelling elderly people: An overview of the literature. *Ageing and Mental Health*, *15*(4), 419–427.

Subject Index

Author Index